My 12-WEEK TRANSFORMATION Journey

Because I DECIDED

with Mariah McCullough

This is

12-WEEK

Journey

BEFORE PHOTO

AFTER PHOTO

START DATE

END DATE

WHY

CONTENTS

Hi there! I'm Mariah and I am honored to be a part of YOUR journey!

Since 2008 I've lost and kept off over 100lb, which I'm so proud of – but take it from me, it wasn't an easy path! I tried so many different diet and exercise plans, most that made me miserable, and none that gave me a sustainable way to transform my body.

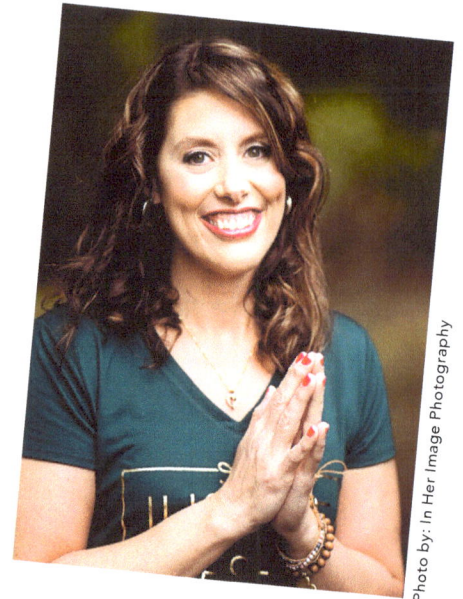

Photo by: In Her Image Photography

My path may not be that different than yours, in fact – I didn't really struggle with my weight growing up, and in fact was an athlete in college. The problems came later, when work and life took over and my health and weight took a back seat. The day I delivered my son, I weighed 275 pounds. I was embarrassed and shocked that I had let my weight balloon up to this amount.

Over 5 years I tried everything from weight-loss pills to excessive exercise, nothing sticking until I realized that successful weight loss and maintenance is less about finding the 'perfect' diet and exercise program, and more about being able to actually stick to something for the long-term. If you think about it, that's where so many of us fail!

My problem was that I wasn't following anything long enough to get lasting results, partly because they all felt like such a struggle. So to solve my weight issues once and for all, I created a system that let me stick to the right way of eating and exercising, and Because I Decided was born.

By learning how low carb eating works, and receiving my support, thousands of women just like you have regained their confidence and hope for the future! They feel energized and happy each and every day, WITHOUT a single thought about how tight their jeans are getting. Not to mention, they still get to enjoy the treats they love without feeling guilt and shame. To date I've helped thousands of woman lose weight while nourishing their bodies and enjoying it, and my goal is to continue helping others to achieve exactly what I've achieved.

(✔)

HAVE YOU DECIDED?

Sound good? Maybe it's time YOU decided.

The First Time I Felt Fat

I remember feeling fat as far back as 8th grade. I was with friends at church playing a clean version of the game "Never Have I Ever". If you don't know how to play the game, basically someone says "Never have I ever…. And then they say something they've never done. The other people playing either fess up to having done it or they have to do a dare.

It was George Duke's turn to go and he said, "Never have I ever weighed 190 pounds" then he stared right at me. I was mortified and began furiously praying that he would not humiliate me. Unfortunately, my prayers weren't answered. When no one raised their hand to say they had ever weighed 190 lbs., George pointed at me and loudly yelled "Mariah has! Mariah has! Look how fat she is!". I was horrified. My face and neck began to burn from my humiliation. All I could do was weakly fumble out that it wasn't true and that I didn't weigh that much.

As soon as I got in the van with my mom and sister to leave church, I started bawling but I was too embarrassed to tell them what happened. When we got home I fled to my room, flung myself on my bed and sobbed the broken-hearted tears of a 13-year-old girl who had been humiliated about her body in front of her friends. My dad was finally able to coax out of me why I was so upset. And as any good father would do, he gave me a huge hug and kiss, told me he loved me and that I was beautiful, that George was a stupid boy, and then gave me step-by-step instructions on how to break his nose (or anyone else's) who ever talked to me like that again.

The truth is, I didn't weigh 190 pounds. I weighed closer to 130. But, regardless of my actual weight, that was a defining moment for me. I was bigger than most of the other girls my age, but I wasn't fat and didn't feel fat until that day. From that moment on, I was acutely aware of my size and how I looked next to all of the skinny 90-pound girls I went to church and school with.

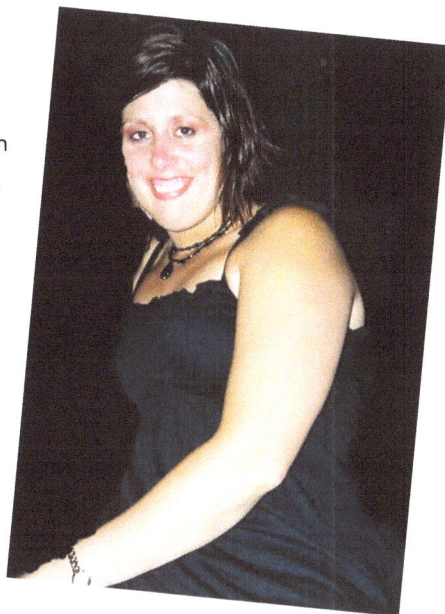

When was the first time you felt like your body wasn't the right size?

I started to hide

I began to wear looser clothing in attempts to hide my body. As the years went by, I continued to carry that shame with me. After college, I started packing on the pounds until I reached an all-time high of 275 pounds on the day I delivered my son. I remember

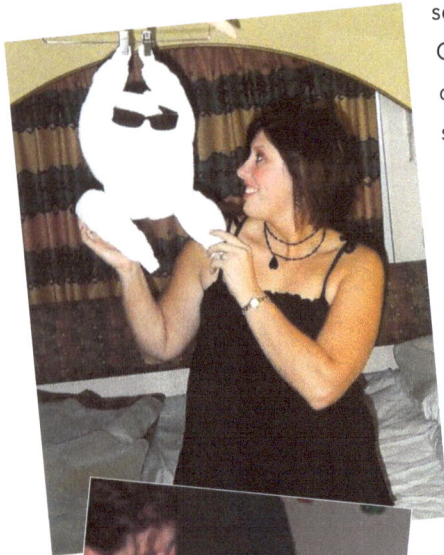

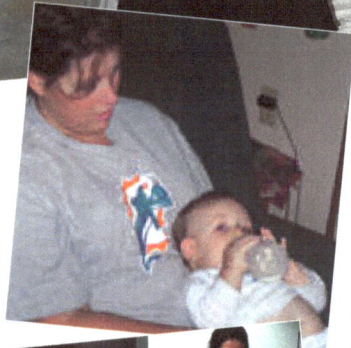

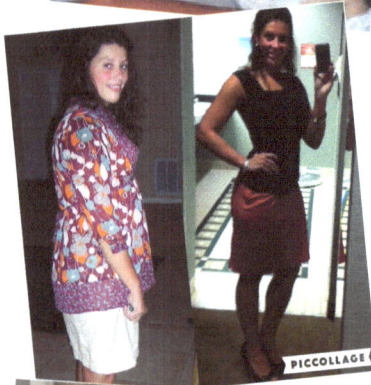

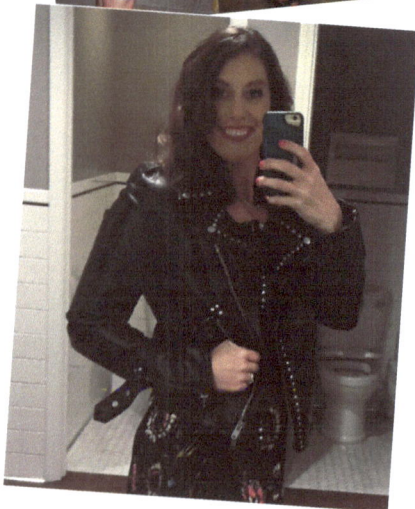

seeing that number on the scale and feeling the same humiliation, I felt when George Duke called me fat. I felt shame at being 25 pounds away from 300. I couldn't believe I had allowed myself to get so fat...so disgusting...so out of shape. I was so disgusted with myself.

As a new mom, there was a message on replay in my mind. It was "you are disgusting. How could you let yourself get so fat? You should be humiliated. Don't let anyone see you. They will see how fat and gross you've become."

And then it happened.

I ran into a nice woman I had known most of my life but hadn't seen in a few years. I saw the shock spread across her face as she looked me up and down realizing who I was. She wasn't being intentionally cruel. That's not her nature. It was an honest reaction to seeing who I'd become. She knew me when I was an athletic 150 pounds and now she was seeing me 100 pounds heavier. And once again, I felt the same heat spread across my face and neck that I felt so many years ago when I was called fat at church in the 8th grade.

After that, I stopped going out in public except to go to work. I refused to go the grocery store. I refused to go to most social events. I refused to have my picture taken and if a picture was taken of me, I cropped myself out of it.

I wanted to disappear from life. I was letting my body hold me back.

Because I decided...

After spending months upon months lying awake at 2:00 am detesting myself and feeling hopeless, I decided I wasn't going out that way. My story wasn't going to end in obesity. I knew I had a long way to go. But I also knew I was the only one who could change my life.

So, on December 28, 2008 I officially started my transformation journey.

I started off doing great. I lost weight following a healthy eating and exercise plan. By the end of the first year, I'd dropped nearly 100 pounds. I was thrilled to fit into regular-sized clothes (goodbye size 22 pants!!). I was excited to be able to get up off of the ground without needing assistance. And I started doing the family grocery shopping again.

I wish I could tell you that it was easy, fast, and that all of my body image issues magically disappeared. But a transformation is more than just about diet and exercise. Because even when you lose the weight, there's still the same woman inside the new body.

The woman who avoids mirrors at all costs terrified at what she will see.

The woman who critically examines her body for flaws

The woman who carries the weight of her secret self-hatred

The woman who masks her pain with big smiles, hollow laughs and secret binges.

The woman who can't accept a compliment about herself because she doesn't think she is deserving of any of them.

The woman who won't ask for help because she doesn't think she is worthy of it.

The woman who secretly feels like she is doomed to be fat and undesirable her entire life.

The woman who feels judging eyes of everyone when she gains 5 lbs.

The woman who places her value as a woman in the way her body looks and in how much it weighs.

The woman who holds herself to unrealistic standards and never feels good enough....

...but all that is about to change!

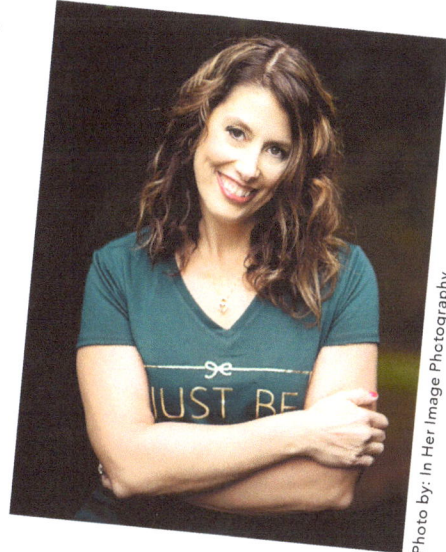

Photo by: In Her Image Photography

> I know this transformation is painful, but you're not falling apart; you're just falling into something different, with a new capacity to be beautiful
>
> —WILLIAM C. HANNAN

FOLLOW ME: f P BecauseIDecided O Because_I_Decided

You are what you eat.

And I'm not talking about food.

What do you tell yourself every day?

What messages are you feeding your mind and soul with?

Are they thoughts based in fear like:

I'm not good enough.

I'm not skinny enough.

I'm not pretty enough.

I'm not enough.

Or do you feed yourself with loving reminders that:

You are enough and that you are worthy of everything your heart desires?

Feed your mind with nourishing messages about yourself and you will be amazed at how you transform.

You in?!

Because I
DECIDED

with Mariah McCullough

These are others who "Decided"

Here are a few of the 6,000+ incredible women who joined the Because I Decided movement and DECIDED to change their lives by changing their bodies. I saved a spot for you to add your picture and would love to feature YOU in future journals.

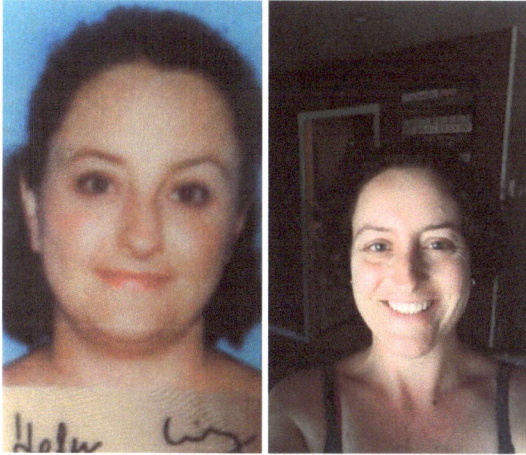

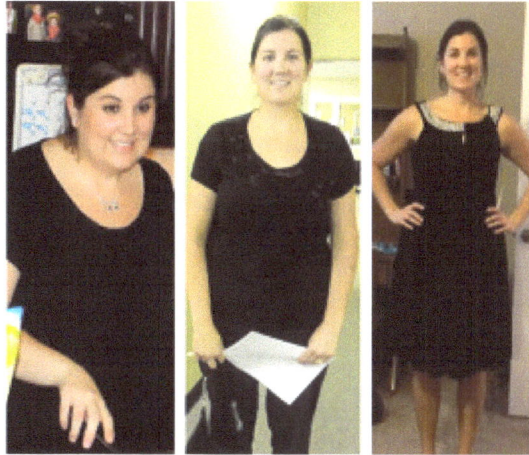

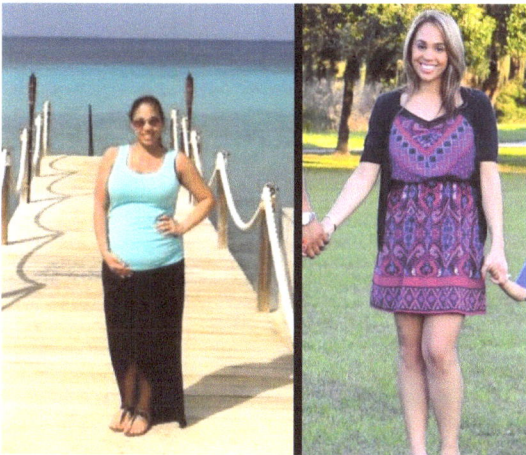

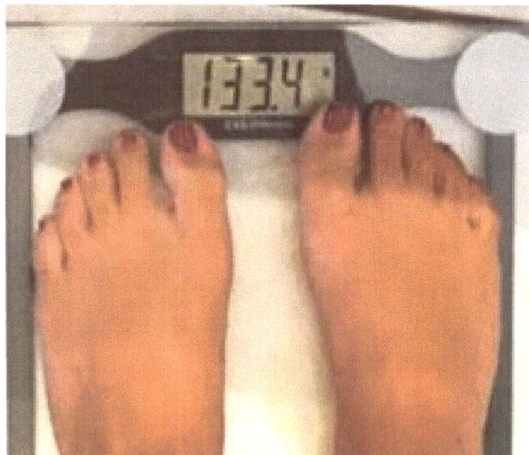

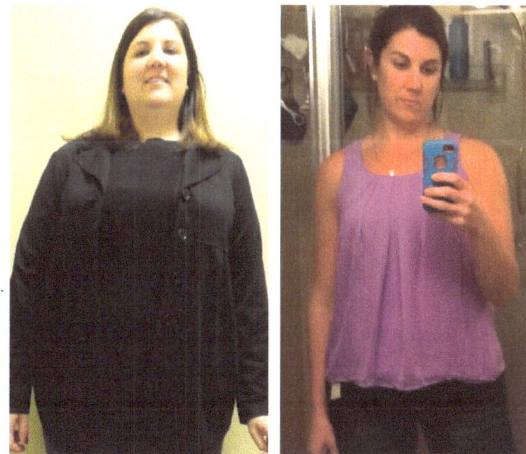

Place for progress picture documentation

FOLLOW ME: BecauseIDecided   Because I Decided

How to
USE THIS
Journal

Because I
DECIDED

with Mariah McCullough

My 90-Day Transformational Journal

90 Days to a Successful Transformation

Congratulations on deciding to change your life. I know you are excited about what lies ahead for you. And you should be! Who you become over the next 90 days will change not just your body but also your mind and your life.

How amazing is it to know that you have the power to completely transform yourself?? **You did the hard part – You DECIDED to change.** You picked this journal, which is the tool that will help you achieve your transformation. All that's left is to consistently show up for yourself over the next 90 days. That's it. You've got this!

This journal was created to be your companion, your roadmap, your place to document your journey during your 90-day transformation so you don't have to guess what you must do, nor do you have to do it alone.

This planner will help you easily track the critical components you need for a successful transformation. Things like eating your veggies, exercise, changes in your body, celebrations, and much more.

I've used this exact process to create my own amazing transformation and lose (and keep off) over 100 pounds. If this process works for me, **I PROMISE it will work for you**.

My 90-Day Transformation Journal contains a goal system, daily, weekly and monthly trackers, and place for you to reflect on your progress. There are also helpful tips, inspirational quotes and more. (You'll find instructions on how to use specific portions of this journal as you go through the journal.)

Go all in for the next 90 days. Be committed to your transformation. Show up every day for yourself; even when you aren't sure if it's worth the effort. Even if you are tired. Even if you doubt yourself. **Commit to showing up EVERY. SINGLE. DAY.**

If you do, I promise you will be amazed at the mind, body and life transformation you will experience.

Because I Decided I transformed my mind, body, and life. Now it's YOUR turn.

Your transformation guide,

Mariah McCullough

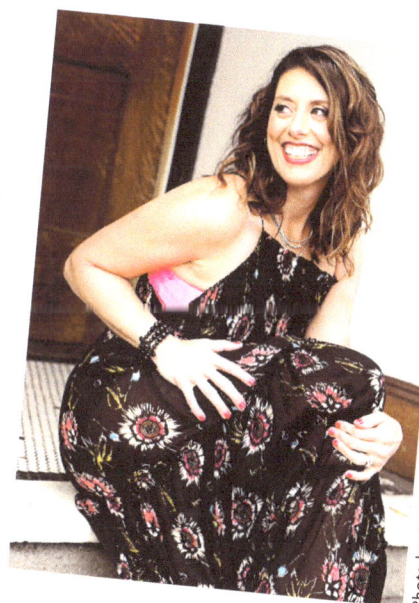

Mariah McCullough

Photo by: In Her Image Photography

This journal was designed to be your companion and your playbook for your 90-Day transformation

In this journal, you will find:

Progress picture

Body composition tracking

Calendars to plan ahead

Tips/Tricks/Strategies

Quick tips

Guidance on:

Controllable vs. non-controllable goals and outcomes

Delaying gratification

Throughout the journal, you'll find further details and definitions that will explain how to track, what controllables and non-controllables are and so much more.

What you won't find in this journal is a specific meal plan to follow. This is because this journal can be used with ANY meal plan you choose. I used it successfully when I ate ultra-low carb, counted calories, counted macros and followed a flexible dieting approach. However, if you are an ultra-low carber, you can use the 10-Day Low Carb Challenge meal plan + template and follow the guidelines in it for your diet. If you joined the My 90-Day Transformation Journey VIP, then you can ask questions about diet in there and once-a- week I'll answer your questions.

In this journal you will find a place for goal setting, daily tracking, milestone tracking, progress pictures, stats, and so much more. As you delve more into the journal, you will read more about each of these things. Use this journal to guide you on your journey and help you create a routine that will lead to your incredible transformation.

QUICK TIP

This isn't a fillable PDF so that means you'll need to print it out. This is intentional. This is to get pen (or pencil) to paper. Science has proven that when you put pen to paper, you're more committed. So print this journal out at your house or send it to Staples to print and bind it and make it your manual for your transformation.

How to measure progress.

The best way to measure your progress is to weigh yourself daily and take progress pictures weekly on the same day and at the same time.

Both your weight and progress pictures help you to measure your progress. Why Weigh?

Knowing your weight is important because it allows you to see if you are trending in the right direction. It also allows you to begin to see how your body responds to stress, lack of sleep, changes in hormones, etc.... As you learn more about your body, fluctuations in weight won't bother you as much because you'll be able to identify whether it's a normal temporary gain or not and adjust accordingly.

But I don't wanna take pics...

I hear you. Trust me. I do. Most people who are at the beginning of their weight-loss journeys don't want to take pictures of themselves. I didn't either. But, I did it anyway and I'm glad I did. It helped me to see progress that I didn't see on the scale or even in the mirror. Progress pictures help you see when your love handles are shrinking, your rear is lifting and your waist is tightening. The scale can't show you those things.

Taking weekly progress pictures is one of my favorite ways to track and see progress because it shows what the scale doesn't; shrinking love handles, slimmer face, and muscles popping out. Whenever I'm serious about making a transformation, I take progress pictures EVERY week and compare them to my starting picture.

THESE ARE MY GO- TO PROGRESS PIC TAKING, COLLAGE MAKING, AND PRIVATE PIC STORING APPS.

AUTO CAM is a self-timer pic taking app. I use to take my pics. Most phones these days have delayed timers, which work fine, but if your phone doesn't, you can use Auto Cam.

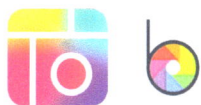

PIC COLLAGE AND BEFUNKY ARE COLLAGE MAKING APPS.
In Pic Collage, you can save previous collages and update weekly. I use this app when I'm updating side by side beginning and current progress pics. BeFunky doesn't store previous versions of collages. Both apps have text writing features and are essentially the same except for the saving of previous versions.

PHOTO VAULT is where I store my progress pics. I set it up to require my fingerprint and 4-digit passcode to unlock. When I started on my fitness journey, I was mortified at the thought of someone seeing a pic of me in a sports bra and pants so I got this app to hide my pics. I continue to use it because it allows me to create folders. I create folders and name them the date of my progress pic and I can easily look at progress pics for any week since April 2013.

PIC COLLAGE APP

This app is great for side-by-side comparisons of your starting picture and your current and/or ending picture. You may want to blow this off because you don't want to take starting pictures, but I PROMISE if you take the pics and follow the program, you will be happy to have your pictures so you can see all of the progress you've made along the way.

HOW TO USE THIS JOURNAL

How to take progress pictures

1. Wear clothing that allows you to see changes in your body like sports bra and workout pants or shorts or a bathing suit
2. Take weekly at the same time in the same place
3. Use app like "Auto Cam" for delayed pic taking so you can take pics on your own.
4. Use an app like "Pic Collage" or "BeFunky" to compare pics and look for progress
5. Compare starting pics to current pics instead of previous week pics to see overall changes
6. Date pics
7. Store in "Photo Vault" app or similar one. This app can be set up to require a password so your progress pics are safe in case a nosy friend (or child) snoops through your phone
8. Celebrate the changes you see in your body!

YOUR ACTION: Pick a day and time to weigh yourself and take progress pictures weekly

PHOTO VAULT APP

This has been my go-to progress picture storage app since 2013. Why? Because you can lock your pics and videos behind a PIN and keep your progress pictures hidden from prying eyes. When I first started taking progress pictures, I was horrified at the thought that someone might get my phone and see my pictures. Being able to lock them away in this app, set my mind at ease. Now I have years of progress pictures to go back and view all in one place and so can you. Download this app and get to storing your progress pics!

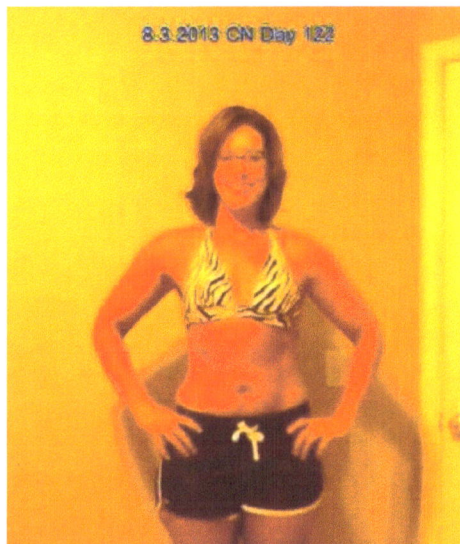

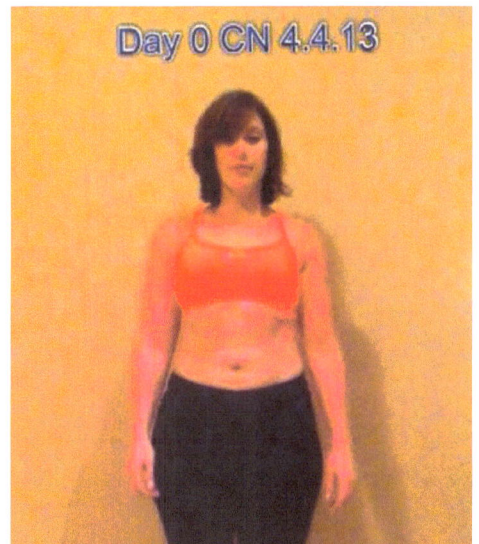

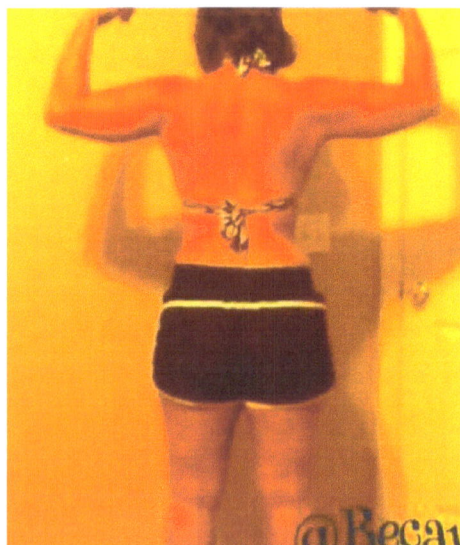

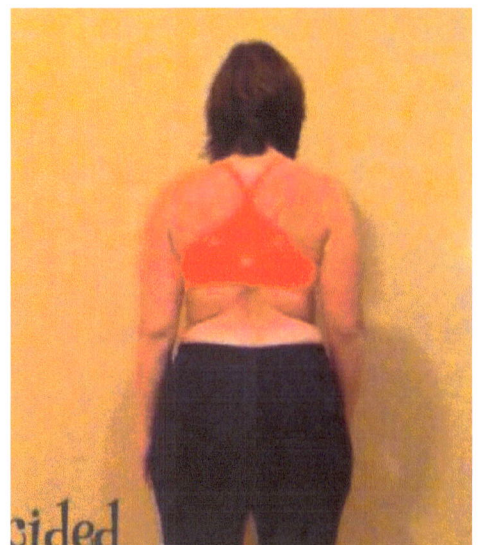

About Controllables and Non-Controllables

Throughout "My 90-Day Transformation Journal" you will primarily focus on setting and tracking controllable outcomes. With weight-loss and physical transformation, there are outcomes we can control ("controllables") and outcomes we can't control ("non-controllables"). Controllables are things like "I will eat 3 servings of green veggies daily" or "I will walk 30 minutes three days a week." These are controllables because you have 100% control on whether you do them or not. On the other hand, non-controllables like "I will lose 3 lbs this week" or "I will lose 1.5" in my waist this week" are outcomes you can't control. Sure, you do things that impact these goals but ultimately you can't control whether you hit them or not. Think about it, how many times have you set a goal to lose let's say 3 lbs in a week, you ate perfectly and exercised daily yet at the end of the week you only lost 1.5 lbs. You likely were frustrated and wanted to quit. Am I right? I know I am because we've all been there. The truth is, our bodies don't lose weight in a linear fashion and if we only focus on non-controllable outcomes then we will be frustrated most of the time. If you focus on controllable outcomes; outcomes that impact non-controllables like weight loss and sizes dropped and celebrate consistency in those areas, then you will have a more joyful journey.

HOW TO TRACK CONTROLLABLES VS NON-CONTROLLABLES

Pick 1–3 things you can "control" related to your diet and 1–2 you can control related to exercise. If you want, you can create 1 non-controllable goal such as number of pounds or inches you want to lose. Keep track of what you stick with, with a simple "1" = Yes and "0" = No. See a sample filled out below.

CONTROLS 1=Y 0=N	S	M	T	W	TH	F	S	TOTAL
1 (DIET)								
Eat 3 cups of green veggies	1	1	0	1	0	1	1	5
2 (DIET)								
Drink 64-oz of water	1	1	1	1	1	1	1	7
3 (DIET)								
Eat 1,800 calories	1	0	1	1	0	1	0	4
1 (EXERCISE)								
Weight train 3 x this week	1	0	1	0	1	0	0	3
2 (EXERCISE)								
Walk for 30 min. 3x this week	0	1	0	1	0	1	0	3
1 (NON-CONTROLLABLE)								
(optional) Lose 1.5lbs		-.25			-.25			-.5

Planning for Life Events

Years ago, when I was stuck in the never-ending cycle of starting a diet on Monday and stopping by the following weekend due to one excuse or another, I realized that there will always be events in life that pop up and serve as excuses to go off track. Things like Mother's Day, birthdays of friends or family, vacations, holidays, and so on. It seemed like every week another celebration would pop up, I wasn't prepared for it and would use it as an excuse to eat all the party foods I could. But, in 2008, weighing 270+ pounds, I decided I'd had enough and that there would always be a reason to celebrate. Instead of playing a victim to events popping up, I decided to take control and plan ahead. The first 90 days, I decided not to partake in any celebrations because I didn't want to put myself in a situation that I wasn't sure I could handle.

After the initial 90 days, when I was stronger, I started to plan out my celebrations. I'd look out 30-90 days ahead and put upcoming celebrations on my calendar. These celebrations were events that I knew would have foods and drinks that weren't part of my normal diet. Once I penciled in the celebrations, I decided which ones I would attend, which ones I would allow myself some treats at and which ones I would attend but stick to my normal eating fare. This allowed me to still enjoy celebrations AND not gain weight. That's what I call a win win!!

Delayed Gratification

Now it's your turn. Use the 3 month blank calendar to write down any celebrations that will occur over the next 90 days. Decide in advance which ones (if any) you will enjoy a treat at and which you will stick to your normal fare. It's also a good time to decide if you should skip the event altogether to help you stay on track. (I'm talking about skipping a work lunch or Happy Hour, not your mom's birthday here!) Update the calendar as frequently as needed. See a sample filled out below.

	MON	TUE	WED	THU	FRI	SAT	SUN
	1	2	3	4	5 *Margarita Happy Hr w/girls*	6	7
	8	9	10	11	12	13	14
October	15	16	17	18	19	20 *Strawberry Shortcake / Mom's BDay*	21
	22	23	24	25	26	27	28
	29	30	31 *Halloween candy- all of it*				

MONTH 1

MAKE A DEAL WITH YOURSELF

Over the next 90 days, choose your transformation over temporary gratification. Write the temporary gratification on your calendar. At the end of your journey, if you want it, then eat it. But, I suspect you won't want it anymore because you will have transformed yourself and your approach to what you indulge in and how often.

Celebrate Your Wins!

For far too many women, successful weight loss is all about the number on the scale. And, if that number goes up (or not down quickly enough), they feel defeated and depressed and often give up. That's not going to happen to you because you are going to learn to recognize and celebrate non-scale victories (NSVs). Non-scale victories (NSVs) are wins you have during your transformation that have nothing to do with your weight. Celebrating NSVs help you notice the progress you're making that isn't necessarily reflected on the scale. Tracking and celebrating progress in a variety of forms can lessen your dependence on the scale and help you mix up your goals. Remember, the scale is simply a measure of your body weight and nothing more. It doesn't tell you your clothes size, inches lost, muscle gained, health gained, etc.

SOME EXAMPLES OF NSV ARE:

· Losing an inch in your waist
· Going down a pant size
· Having enough energy to play with your child or grandchild
· Feeling good in your clothes
· Fitting in the rollercoaster seat
· Finishing a 5k
· Eating according to your goals instead of circumstances
· Going to the gym and working out 3x's during the week

It's important to recognize changes, even if you consider them small as they are happening. If you focus on NSVs, the pounds will take care of themselves (promise!). You'll realize that you're changing behaviors and making better choices that will last you a lifetime at a healthy weight. Use the space below to write down NSVs.

HERE ARE A FEW EXAMPLES OF SOME WAYS YOU CAN CELEBRATE AS YOU HIT MILESTONES ALONG YOUR JOURNEY.

There are hundreds of ways you can celebrate. Start making your own list. You can group your "celebration wish list" by cost or by what you can choose from when you hit a certain milestone. It's really up to you on how you want to make this work for you!

LOW OR NO COST OR WHEN YOU HIT MILESTONE 1	MEDIUM COST OR WHEN YOU HIT MILESTONE 2	HIGH COST OR WHEN YOU HIT MILESTONE 3
Manicure	Massage	FitBit
Pedicure	New workout outfit	Get professional pictures taken
Hot bubble bath	New tennis shoes	New wardrobe
New book	New outift	Weekend away
Try a new workout class	New purse	Beach trip
See a movie with a friend	New heels	Spa day
	Date night	New camera to take pictures of you in your rocking new clothes
		iWatch

How-to Use This Page

This is where you'll assess how you did during the previous month, identify what you need to tweak to have better success and set your goals for the coming month.

1. What's gone well for you this month?

2. What are some wins you've experienced? *(No win is too small. If you picked chicken over pizza, that's a win! If you lost 1" off of your waist, that's a win. Take a moment to think about your wins and write them below.)*

3. What are some areas you've struggled with? *Can you identify the specific reason you struggled? For example, you might have blown it 4 days when you got home from work. You might think you blew it because you lack will power and gave in to eating chips and dip for dinner instead of veggies and chicken, but, if you really look at it, you might see that you gave in to chips and dip because you: didn't have your dinner prepped ahead of time so you didn't want to wait to eat and you waited too long between meals. If you can identify why you went off course, then you'll be empowered to prevent it in the future.*

4. Take a look back at your weekly check-ins and your controllable vs. uncontrollable chart. *Can you see any correlations between your progress and what your charts are showing you?*

5. What can you focus on this week to make sure you continue to see results?

6. What do you need to adjust for the next month?

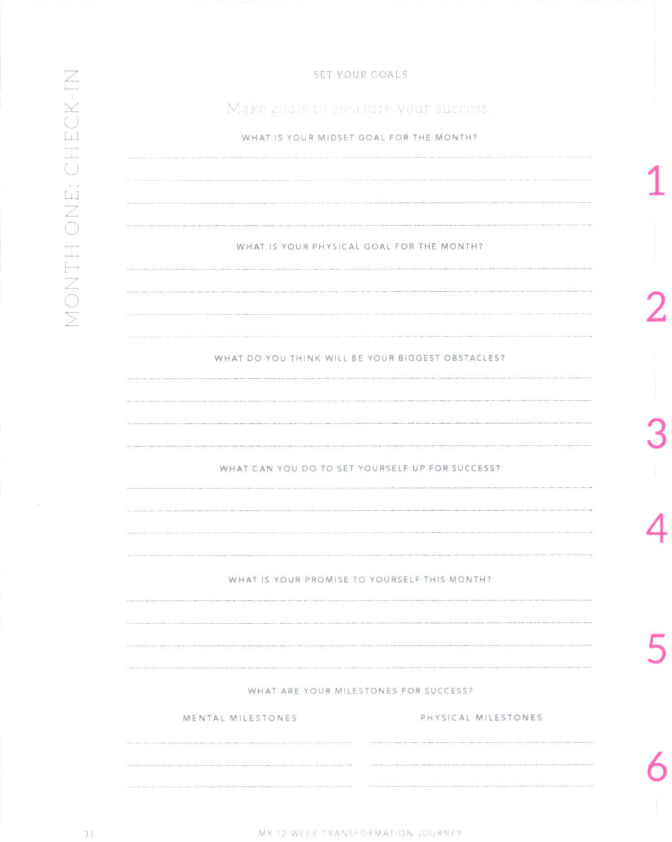

Sidebar panel (Month One: Check-In):

MONTH ONE: CHECK-IN

SET YOUR GOALS

Make goals to measure your success.

WHAT IS YOUR MINDSET GOAL FOR THE MONTH? — 1

WHAT IS YOUR PHYSICAL GOAL FOR THE MONTH? — 2

WHAT DO YOU THINK WILL BE YOUR BIGGEST OBSTACLES? — 3

WHAT CAN YOU DO TO SET YOURSELF UP FOR SUCCESS? — 4

WHAT IS YOUR PROMISE TO YOURSELF THIS MONTH? — 5

WHAT ARE YOUR MILESTONES FOR SUCCESS?

MENTAL MILESTONES   PHYSICAL MILESTONES — 6

MY 12 WEEK TRANSFORMATION JOURNEY

(✓)

THINGS TO KEEP IN MIND

Did you know that pre-period water weight can range from half a pound to 10 pounds, usually averaging five pounds for most women? This is due to the hormone progesterone. Once you start your period, progesterone drops and your body releases all of the water it was holding. This is important for you to pay attention to and to start tracking so that you don't freak out if your weight increases in the days leading up to your period. Instead, you'll know how your body works and won't feel frustrated or discouraged if you see the scale go up prior to your period starting. You'll know that it's a temporary gain and that your weight will stabilize once your period starts.

How-to Use These Pages

Each week, you'll set your controllable and non-controllable outcome goals. You have space for up to 6 outcomes, but you don't have to use that many. *See page 17 for an example.* There were many weeks when I had 2 diet-related controllable outcome goals and 1 exercise controllable outcome goal and that's it. Those weeks tended to be better for me because I laser focused on 3 simple things and made sure I did them every day.

AT THE END OF EVERY WEEK, YOU WILL:

Look back to your previous week check in to review your controllables and non-controllables for the week. Give yourself a "1" if you completed your goal and a "0" if you didn't. Tally up your points for the week. This will show you how you did for the week.

1. Take a front, side and back progress picture, weigh yourself and measure yourself and record your progress on your tracker.

2. Next, write a short summary about your week. Include what went well, any challenges you faced and how you overcame them. Rate your week on a scale of 1 to 10 with 1 being sucky and 10 being outstanding and rate

yourself on Mental Focus, Commitment, Diet and Exercise.

3. Write your controllable and non-controllable outcome goals for the coming week.

4. Prep for the week ahead, and make note of what you can improve upon this coming week.

REMINDER

You will do this every week over the next 90 days. You may want to skip this step. Don't. It's one of the most important factors for staying on track because it holds you accountable for your results.

WEEK 1: CHECK IN

YOU CAN'T MEASURE WHAT YOU DON'T TRACK

FROM / / TO / /

PROGRESS PIC

PROGRESS PIC

1

STATS

	MEASURE	LOSS/GAIN		MEASURE	LOSS/GAIN
BUST			L HIGH		
WAIST			R ARM		
HIPS			L ARM		
R THIGH			WEIGHT		

MIND MAP

WHAT DO YOU HAVE TO OVERCOME THIS WEEK?

2

RATE YOUR DEDICATION ON A SCALE OF 1 TO 10										
MENTAL FOCUS	1	2	3	4	5	6	7	8	9	10
COMMITMENT	1	2	3	4	5	6	7	8	9	10
DIET	1	2	3	4	5	6	7	8	9	10
EXERCISE	1	2	3	4	5	6	7	8	9	10

MY 12 WEEK TRANSFORMATION JOURNEY

WEEK 2: SET UP FOR SUCCESS

PLAN FOR SUCCESS

CONTROLLABLES VS NON CONTROLLABLES

CONTROLS 1=Y 0=N	S	M	T	W	TH	F	S	TOTAL
1 (DIET)								
2 (DIET)								
3 (DIET)								
1 (EXERCISE)								
2 (EXERCISE)								
1 (NON-CONTROLLABLE)								

3

MAKE IT HAPPEN

PREPARATION	GOALS
MEAL PREP	MILESTONE 1
SCHEDULE DIET CONTROLS	MILESTONE 2
SCHEDULE MOVEMENT CONTROLS	MILESTONE 3

WHAT CAN YOU IMPROVE UPON FOR THIS COMING WEEK?

I may not be there yet, but I am closer than I was yesterday

4

MY 12 WEEK TRANSFORMATION JOURNEY

How-to Use These Pages

This should be short and sweet. You can either check in as you complete an item, or you can take 5-10 minutes at the end of every day to track. Every day track your controllables and non-controllables on your weekly set-up page. Give yourself a "1" if you did it and a "0" if you didn't.

1. In the daily check-in section, you will find space to track your meals, workout, and water. It's up to you if you want to track it in your journal or in an app. There are benefits to both.

2. Jot down anything that went well, any challenges you faced and inspiration for tomorrow. Give yourself and overall performance score of 1-10 with 1 being sucky and 10 being AH-MAZING.

3. Saturday and Sunday do not have as much to track, but enough to keep you on track!

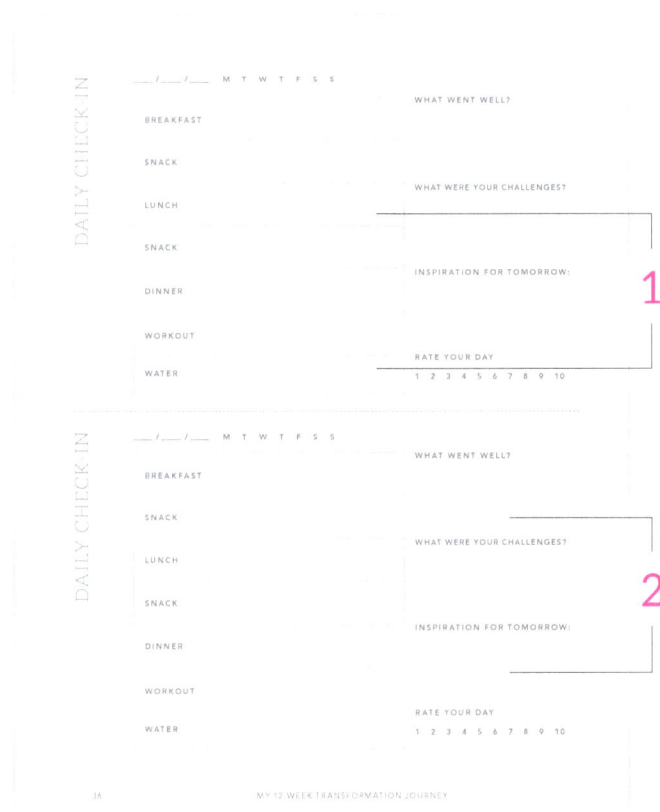

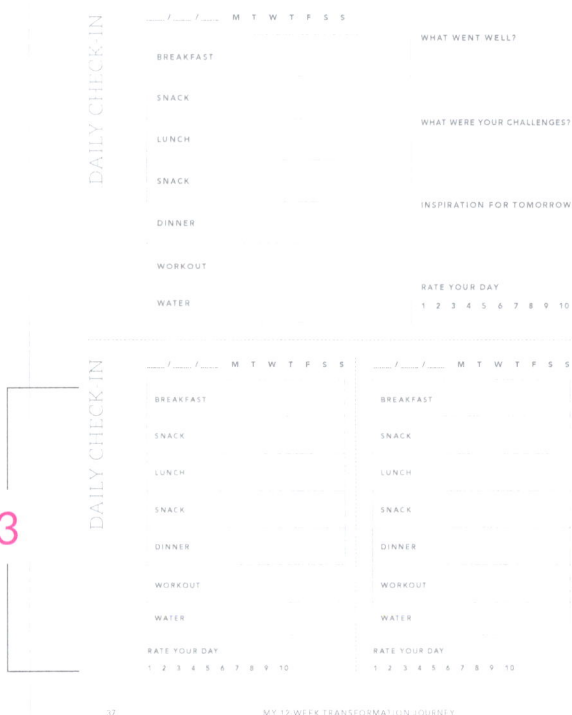

DAILY CHECK IN

___/___/___   M T W T F S S

BREAKFAST

SNACK

LUNCH

SNACK

DINNER

WORKOUT

WATER

WHAT WENT WELL?

WHAT WERE YOUR CHALLENGES?

INSPIRATION FOR TOMORROW:

RATE YOUR DAY
1 2 3 4 5 6 7 8 9 10

1

DAILY CHECK IN

___/___/___   M T W T F S S

BREAKFAST

SNACK

LUNCH

SNACK

DINNER

WORKOUT

WATER

WHAT WENT WELL?

WHAT WERE YOUR CHALLENGES?

INSPIRATION FOR TOMORROW:

RATE YOUR DAY
1 2 3 4 5 6 7 8 9 10

2

DAILY CHECK IN

___/___/___   M T W T F S S

BREAKFAST

SNACK

LUNCH

SNACK

DINNER

WORKOUT

WATER

WHAT WENT WELL?

WHAT WERE YOUR CHALLENGES?

INSPIRATION FOR TOMORROW:

RATE YOUR DAY
1 2 3 4 5 6 7 8 9 10

DAILY CHECK IN

___/___/___   M T W T F S S

BREAKFAST

SNACK

LUNCH

SNACK

DINNER

WORKOUT

WATER

RATE YOUR DAY
1 2 3 4 5 6 7 8 9 10

___/___/___   M T W T F S S

BREAKFAST

SNACK

LUNCH

SNACK

DINNER

WORKOUT

WATER

RATE YOUR DAY
1 2 3 4 5 6 7 8 9 10

3

TRACK WITH PAPER OR APP?

- The benefit of tracking it in your journal is you can see everything in one place and when you look back over your 90 days, you'll be able to see exactly what you ate and how you exercised to create the transformation you created.

- The benefit of tracking through and app is that it's easier for some people.

- Ultimately, pick whichever method works for you and run with it.

Tools, Tricks, and Strategies

Throughout the journal, you'll find tips, tricks and strategies sprinkled on the pages. These are things that I've used along my journey that you may find helpful on yours. Use the ones that work for you and forget about the ones that aren't appealing to you. Remember, this is your journey and you have to make tips, tricks and strategies work for you.

MY FITNESS PAL (MFP) – this is a meal/macro tracker. This one is great because it's free, you can adjust your macros to fit your preferences and you can share your food diary with others. Just make sure you double check the nutritional information on the food in their database. They are entered by users and may contain errors.

HAPPY SCALE – There are thousands of ways to track your weight, but I'm in love with IOS app, Happy Scale. I love it because it's simple; enter your goal weight, date you'd like to achieve that weight and the number of milestones you want set up along the way. Enter your weight (I recommend daily) and the app gives predictions on when you'll reach your next milestone and your final goal. It also creates a simple graph to show your weight loss progress. Plus, you can create a PIN to make your data private!

AVATAR NUTRITION – This is for you if you want to do flexible dieting but have no clue how to figure out your macros. Avatar Nutrition is comprised of PhDs, nutritionists and athletes who created a system that takes the guesswork out of figuring out your macros and utilizes software to adjust your macros based on your results. It's $9.99 per month which is significantly cheaper than hiring a personal trainer or nutritionist to figure out your macros for you and it's a lot easier than doing it yourself.

DAYS UNTIL (IOS APP) – This date allows you to enter a date you want to accomplish a goal by and it will track down with "days until" the event. I use this every time I'm serious about transforming because it keeps me focused and on track knowing that I only have X days to transform.

GYMBOSS APP – This is an interval timer app that allows you to program interval timers that work for you and your workout. You can use it for running, HIIT, EMOM (every minute on the minute workouts), CrossFit and more. It's free and a great addition to your workout.

INSTANT POT (OR ANOTHER PRESSURE COOKER) – Great tool to make dinner in a hurry.

My go-to chicken recipes:

1 cup of chicken broth + frozen chicken breasts or tenders and cook on poultry for 15-20 minutes

1 jar salsa + 1 cup water + frozen chicken breasts or tender and cook on poultry for 15-20 minutes. The chicken falls apart and is delicious!

TRAVEL TIP

Did you know that you can freeze liquids such as water or unsweetened almond milk and use them to keep your food cool when you travel on airplanes? When going through security, take the bottles out of your bag and place them in their own container so security doesn't have to search your bag. As long as the fluids are frozen, you'll be able to take them through with no problem. As an added bonus, once the solids defrost, you have some ready-to-drink water and/or almond milk.

KITCHEN SCALE – This is a must if you want to accurately account for what you're putting in your mouth. Get in the habit of weighing what you eat. Most people significantly under-estimate how much they're eating and get frustrated when they don't lose weight. Don't let that be you. Get a digital kitchen scale. Weigh your food. Lose weight!

CALENDAR & STICKERS – There's something very powerful about putting pen to paper (or in this case calendar), writing your goals and tracking your progress. Put the current month's calendar where you can look at it every morning when you wake up and at night before bed. At the top of it write three goals for the month (complete every workout as scheduled, eat three cups of veggies, etc…) and put a slash and/or sticker on every day you successfully completed your goals.

Pic Collage app – This app is great for side-by-side comparisons of your starting picture and your current and/or ending picture. You may want to blow this off because you don't want to take starting pictures, but I PROMISE if you take the pics and follow the program, you will be happy to have your pictures so you can see all of the progress you've made along the way.

Photo Vault app – this has been my go-to progress picture storage app since 2013. Why? Because you can lock your pics and videos behind a PIN and keep your progress pictures hidden from prying eyes. When I first started taking progress pictures, I was horrified at the thought that someone might get my phone and see my pictures. Being able to lock them away in this app, set my mind at ease. Now I have years of progress pictures to go back and view all in one place and so can you. Download this app and get to storing your progress pics!

✔

TRAVEL TIP

Want to workout on the road but won't have access to a gym? Buy some workout bands and download some band and bodyweight workouts. You can get an amazing workout with bands and your bodyweight. If you're looking for a workout plan that involves bands, check out Fit Thrive's 12-Week Bodyweight and Band Program.

Your Journey
STARTS NOW!

Because I
DECIDED

with Mariah McCullough

YOUR STORY

So what's holding you back?

What stories from the past are holding you back from being the best version of yourself today?

No matter what method, diet or technique you decide on to transform your weight and your life, the most important tool you have on your path to success is your mind. Without a shift in your mind and how you view yourself, it will be difficult to successfully transform. That's why "My 90-Day Transformation Journey" contains a "Mind" focus along with a "Body" and "Life" focus.

If you only focus on changing your weight or your size and don't do any changes internally, you're likely to struggle to reach your ultimate goal. Even though it may be hard to counteract those negative thoughts that may have been with you for many years, take it from me, you can do it! The first step is deciding to start your transformation journey with a positive mindset, and whenever those negative voices in your head start their talking, use your inner strength to banish them. Remember that you're not alone, and with the support I'm going to give you and your commitment to a positive mindset, your inner strength will get stronger and stronger every day!

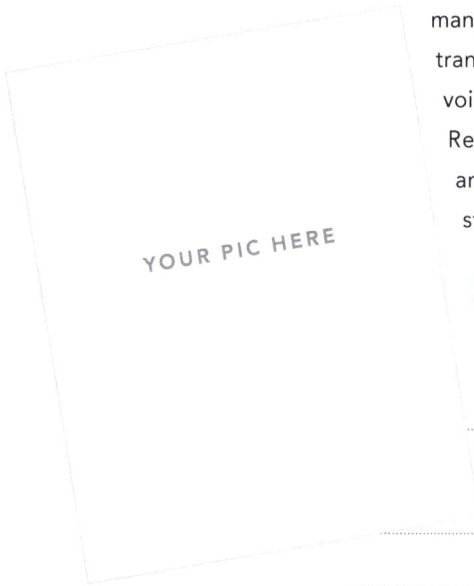

Share your story - what has been holding you back?

YOUR PIC HERE

QUICK TIP

To take the best progress pics, have someone else take them for you. Stand in front of a simple background, or blank wall. If you need to take your own pics, try to take them with a photo timer app.

YOUR ACTION

Pick a day and time to weigh yourself and take progress pictures weekly.

and Why Now...

Do it for the woman you want to become.

Do it so you can finally know what it's like to be comfortable in your own skin.

Do it for the feeling you get when you comfortably fit in those size 8 jeans.

Do it so you can take all of the selfies/pictures you want and LIKE who you see.

Do it so you can rock your swimsuit.

Do it because you only get one chance at this life and you're tired of living on the sidelines.

Make your declarations and commit to why you're going to do it now!

Do it _____

Do it _____

Do it _____

Do it _____

Do it _____

Do it _____

Create a contract with yourself:

"BECAUSE I DECIDED, I WILL TRANSFORM MY MIND, BODY AND LIFE"

_____   _____
Signature   Date

GET BACK IN THE GAME TODAY!

Stop sitting on the sidelines of life due to your weight or body image issues.

Month 1

Michiele's Story

" I started and stopped diets more times than I can count. I was always preparing to start a new diet on Monday. I'd do good for a while, but then I'd end up going out with friends, indulging in a few too many drinks at Happy Hour or honestly just lose focus on what I was trying to accomplish, and I'd give up. I'm a mom of three and I used to feel so sluggish and annoyed with everything I had to deal with as a parent. Things I should have been finding joy in. Things like playing with my kids, going on walks with my family, dancing with them and so much more.

When my kids wanted me to play with them, I didn't want to because I was always so tired. I felt so guilty. I wanted to do better for my family. I wanted to look sexy for my husband. I wanted to feel better for myself. I was tired of constantly starting and stopping a diet and not getting lasting results. I knew I had to do something to change.

With Mariah's guidance, I realized that I had to make lifestyle changes if I wanted to lose weight and keep it off. I had to stop starting and stopping diet after diet and be consistent with my efforts. I DECIDED that I was all in, so I picked an eating plan (low carb worked for me!) and followed the process that Mariah outlined for me. At first, I wasn't sure about the "process" because I had only ever paid attention to diet and exercise before. But, I saw firsthand the transformation Mariah made following her process, so I put my trust in her and did everything she told me to do.

With her help and my decision to stick with it, I lost over 30 pounds and got down to my pre-baby weight (YES!!). I exercise and eat better. My confidence has sky-rocketed. I love going on walks with my family, shopping for cute outfits, and dancing with my husband.

The best part about all of this is now this is just a way of life. No more staring a new diet on Monday! "

MARIAH'S WORDS:

I'm sure you can relate to Michiele's story. We've all been there; too tired to play with our kids, feeling guilty because we are too tired to play with our kids and beating ourselves up because we start and stop a new diet every week. Michiele knew she had to do something different. She trusted me and my process to help her and guide her through her transformation. As a result, she lost over 30 pounds and a ton of inches, but more importantly she gained energy and confidence to start living life again. She and her family are so happy she decided to change.

As you start on your own transformation journey, trust the process because it works. Decide to do it for the full 90 days. You will be so happy that you did.

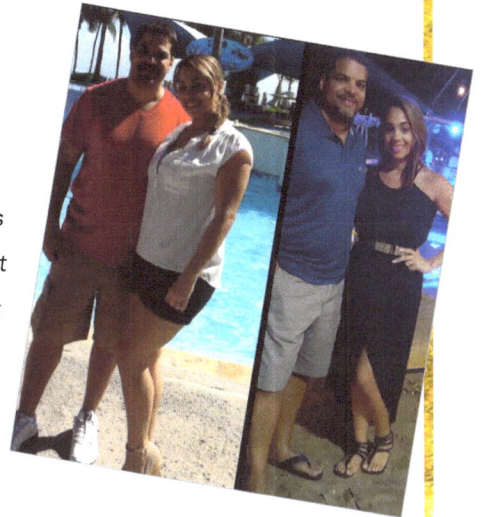

Tips for taking body measurements

1. *Keep the length of the measuring tape parallel to the floor at all times.*

2. *Pull the tape snug, but not so tightly that it squeezes your body.*

3. *Measurements taken around the neck, buttocks, thighs, calves, biceps and forearm should be taken around the largest circumference.*

bust

arms

waist

hips

thighs

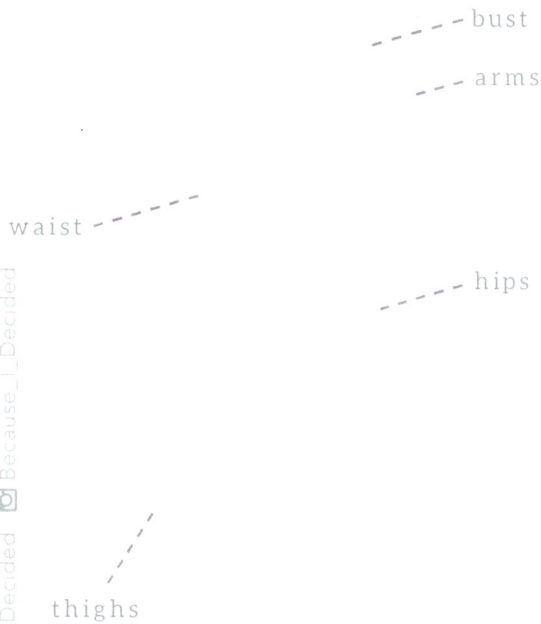

MONTH 1	WK 1	WK 2	WK 3	WK 4	TOTAL +/-
BUST					
WAIST					
HIPS					
R THIGH					
L HIGH					
R ARM					
L ARM					
WEIGHT					

MONTH 2	WK 1	WK 2	WK 3	WK 4	TOTAL +/-
BUST					
WAIST					
HIPS					
R THIGH					
L HIGH					
R ARM					
L ARM					
WEIGHT					

MONTH 3	WK 1	WK 2	WK 3	WK 4	TOTAL +/-
BUST					
WAIST					
HIPS					
R THIGH					
L HIGH					
R ARM					
L ARM					
WEIGHT					

TRACK SPECIAL DAYS THAT MIGHT CHALLENGE YOU SO YOU CAN BE PREPARED

MON	TUE	WED	THU	FRI	SAT	SUN

MONTH 1

MON	TUE	WED	THU	FRI	SAT	SUN

MONTH 2

MON	TUE	WED	THU	FRI	SAT	SUN

MONTH 3

SET YOUR GOALS

Make goals to measure your success.

WHAT IS YOUR MIDSET GOAL FOR THE MONTH?

....

....

....

....

WHAT IS YOUR PHYSICAL GOAL FOR THE MONTH?

....

....

....

....

WHAT DO YOU THINK WILL BE YOUR BIGGEST OBSTACLES?

....

....

....

....

WHAT CAN YOU DO TO SET YOURSELF UP FOR SUCCESS?

....

....

....

....

WHAT IS YOUR PROMISE TO YOURSELF THIS MONTH?

....

....

....

....

WHAT ARE YOUR MILESTONES FOR SUCCESS?

MENTAL MILESTONES	PHYSICAL MILESTONES
....	....
....	....
....	....

YOU CAN'T MEASURE WHAT YOU DON'T TRACK

FROM___ /___ /___   TO___ /___ /___

```
+----------------------+      +----------------------+
|                      |      |                      |
|                      |      |                      |
|                      |      |                      |
|     PROGRESS PIC     |      |     PROGRESS PIC     |
|                      |      |                      |
|                      |      |                      |
|                      |      |                      |
+----------------------+      +----------------------+
```

STATS

	MEASURE	LOSS/GAIN		MEASURE	LOSS/GAIN
BUST			L HIGH		
WAIST			R ARM		
HIPS			L ARM		
R THIGH			WEIGHT		

MIND MAP

WHAT DO YOU HAVE TO OVERCOME THIS WEEK?

....

....

....

RATE YOUR DEDICATION	MENTAL FOCUS	1 2 3 4 5 6 7 8 9 10
	COMMITMENT	1 2 3 4 5 6 7 8 9 10
	DIET	1 2 3 4 5 6 7 8 9 10
ON A SCALE OF 1 TO 10	EXERCISE	1 2 3 4 5 6 7 8 9 10

PLAN FOR SUCCESS

CONTROLLABLES VS NON-CONTROLLABLES

CONTROLS 1=Y 0=N	S	M	T	W	TH	F	S	TOTAL
1 (DIET)								
2 (DIET)								
3 (DIET)								
1 (EXERCISE)								
2 (EXERCISE)								
1 (NON-CONTROLLABLE)								

- - - - - - - - - - - - - - - - - - - MAKE IT HAPPEN - - - - - - - - - - - - - - - - - - -

PREPARATION

MEAL PREP

SCHEDULE DIET CONTROLS

SCHEDULE MOVEMENT CONTROLS

GOALS

MILESTONE 1

MILESTONE 2

MILESTONE 3

WHAT CAN YOU DO TO STAY ON TRACK?

I may not be there yet, but I am closer than I was yesterday.

.... / .... / ....   M   T   W   T   F   S   S

BREAKFAST	
SNACK	
LUNCH	
SNACK	
DINNER	
WORKOUT	
WATER	

WHAT WENT WELL?

WHAT WERE YOUR CHALLENGES?

INSPIRATION FOR TOMORROW:

RATE YOUR DAY

1   2   3   4   5   6   7   8   9   10

.... / .... / ....   M   T   W   T   F   S   S

BREAKFAST	
SNACK	
LUNCH	
SNACK	
DINNER	
WORKOUT	
WATER	

WHAT WENT WELL?

WHAT WERE YOUR CHALLENGES?

INSPIRATION FOR TOMORROW:

RATE YOUR DAY

1   2   3   4   5   6   7   8   9   10

DAILY CHECK-IN

.... / .... / .... M T W T F S S

	WHAT WENT WELL?
BREAKFAST	
SNACK	
LUNCH	WHAT WERE YOUR CHALLENGES?
SNACK	
DINNER	INSPIRATION FOR TOMORROW:
WORKOUT	
WATER	RATE YOUR DAY
	1 2 3 4 5 6 7 8 9 10

DAILY CHECK-IN

.... / .... / .... M T W T F S S

	WHAT WENT WELL?
BREAKFAST	
SNACK	
LUNCH	WHAT WERE YOUR CHALLENGES?
SNACK	
DINNER	INSPIRATION FOR TOMORROW:
WORKOUT	
WATER	RATE YOUR DAY
	1 2 3 4 5 6 7 8 9 10

.... / .... / ....   M T W T F S S

| BREAKFAST |
| SNACK |
| LUNCH |
| SNACK |
| DINNER |
| WORKOUT |
| WATER |

WHAT WENT WELL?

WHAT WERE YOUR CHALLENGES?

INSPIRATION FOR TOMORROW:

RATE YOUR DAY

1   2   3   4   5   6   7   8   9   10

.... / .... / ....   M T W T F S S

| BREAKFAST |
| SNACK |
| LUNCH |
| SNACK |
| DINNER |
| WORKOUT |
| WATER |

RATE YOUR DAY

1   2   3   4   5   6   7   8   9   10

.... / .... / ....   M T W T F S S

| BREAKFAST |
| SNACK |
| LUNCH |
| SNACK |
| DINNER |
| WORKOUT |
| WATER |

RATE YOUR DAY

1   2   3   4   5   6   7   8   9   10

YOU CAN'T MEASURE WHAT YOU DON'T TRACK

FROM ___ / ___ / ___   TO___ / ___ / __

PROGRESS PIC

PROGRESS PIC

STATS

	MEASURE	LOSS/GAIN		MEASURE	LOSS/GAIN
BUST			L HIGH		
WAIST			R ARM		
HIPS			L ARM		
R THIGH			WEIGHT		

MIND MAP

WHAT DO YOU HAVE TO OVERCOME THIS WEEK?

....

....

....

....

RATE YOUR
DEDICATION
ON A SCALE OF 1 TO 10

MENTAL FOCUS	1	2	3	4	5	6	7	8	9	10
COMMITMENT	1	2	3	4	5	6	7	8	9	10
DIET	1	2	3	4	5	6	7	8	9	10
EXERCISE	1	2	3	4	5	6	7	8	9	10

PLAN FOR SUCCESS

CONTROLLABLES VS NON-CONTROLLABLES

CONTROLS 1=Y 0=N	S	M	T	W	TH	F	S	TOTAL
1 (DIET)								
2 (DIET)								
3 (DIET)								
1 (EXERCISE)								
2 (EXERCISE)								
1 (NON-CONTROLLABLE)								

- - - - - - - - - - MAKE IT HAPPEN - - - - - - - - - -

PREPARATION	GOALS
MEAL PREP	MILESTONE 1
SCHEDULE DIET CONTROLS	MILESTONE 2
SCHEDULE MOVEMENT CONTROLS	MILESTONE 3

WHAT CAN YOU IMPROVE UPON FOR THIS COMING WEEK?

I may not be there yet, but I am closer than I was yesterday.

FOLLOW ME: f P Because_I_Decided Because_I_Decided

DAILY CHECK-IN

.... / .... / ....   M   T   W   T   F   S   S

BREAKFAST	
SNACK	
LUNCH	
SNACK	
DINNER	
WORKOUT	
WATER	

WHAT WENT WELL?

WHAT WERE YOUR CHALLENGES?

INSPIRATION FOR TOMORROW:

RATE YOUR DAY

1   2   3   4   5   6   7   8   9   10

DAILY CHECK-IN

.... / .... / ....   M   T   W   T   F   S   S

BREAKFAST	
SNACK	
LUNCH	
SNACK	
DINNER	
WORKOUT	
WATER	

WHAT WENT WELL?

WHAT WERE YOUR CHALLENGES?

INSPIRATION FOR TOMORROW:

RATE YOUR DAY

1   2   3   4   5   6   7   8   9   10

.... / .... / ....   M   T   W   T   F   S   S

| BREAKFAST |
| SNACK |
| LUNCH |
| SNACK |
| DINNER |
| WORKOUT |
| WATER |

WHAT WENT WELL?

WHAT WERE YOUR CHALLENGES?

INSPIRATION FOR TOMORROW:

RATE YOUR DAY

1   2   3   4   5   6   7   8   9   10

.... / .... / ....   M   T   W   T   F   S   S

| BREAKFAST |
| SNACK |
| LUNCH |
| SNACK |
| DINNER |
| WORKOUT |
| WATER |

WHAT WENT WELL?

WHAT WERE YOUR CHALLENGES?

INSPIRATION FOR TOMORROW:

RATE YOUR DAY

1   2   3   4   5   6   7   8   9   10

DAILY CHECK-IN

.... / .... / ....   M T W T F S S

BREAKFAST	
SNACK	
LUNCH	
SNACK	
DINNER	
WORKOUT	
WATER	

WHAT WENT WELL?

WHAT WERE YOUR CHALLENGES?

INSPIRATION FOR TOMORROW:

RATE YOUR DAY

1   2   3   4   5   6   7   8   9   10

DAILY CHECK-IN

.... / .... / ....   M T W T F S S

BREAKFAST	
SNACK	
LUNCH	
SNACK	
DINNER	
WORKOUT	
WATER	

WHAT WENT WELL?

WHAT WERE YOUR CHALLENGES?

INSPIRATION FOR TOMORROW:

RATE YOUR DAY

1   2   3   4   5   6   7   8   9   10

.... / .... / ....   M   T   W   T   F   S   S

BREAKFAST	
SNACK	
LUNCH	
SNACK	
DINNER	
WORKOUT	
WATER	

WHAT WENT WELL?

WHAT WERE YOUR CHALLENGES?

INSPIRATION FOR TOMORROW:

RATE YOUR DAY

1   2   3   4   5   6   7   8   9   10

YOU CAN'T MEASURE WHAT YOU DON'T TRACK

FROM ___ / ___ / ___ TO ___ / ___ / ___

PROGRESS PIC

PROGRESS PIC

STATS

	MEASURE	LOSS/GAIN		MEASURE	LOSS/GAIN
BUST			L HIGH		
WAIST			R ARM		
HIPS			L ARM		
R THIGH			WEIGHT		

MIND MAP

WHAT DO YOU HAVE TO OVERCOME THIS WEEK?

....
....
....
....

RATE YOUR DEDICATION ON A SCALE OF 1 TO 10											
MENTAL FOCUS	1	2	3	4	5	6	7	8	9	10
COMMITMENT	1	2	3	4	5	6	7	8	9	10
DIET	1	2	3	4	5	6	7	8	9	10
EXERCISE	1	2	3	4	5	6	7	8	9	10

PLAN FOR SUCCESS

CONTROLLABLES VS NON-CONTROLLABLES

CONTROLS 1=Y 0=N	S	M	T	W	TH	F	S	TOTAL
1 (DIET)								
2 (DIET)								
3 (DIET)								
1 (EXERCISE)								
2 (EXERCISE)								
1 (NON-CONTROLLABLE)								

- - - - - - - - - - - - MAKE IT HAPPEN - - - - - - - - - - - -

PREPARATION
MEAL PREP

SCHEDULE DIET CONTROLS

SCHEDULE MOVEMENT CONTROLS

GOALS
MILESTONE 1

MILESTONE 2

MILESTONE 3

WHAT CAN YOU IMPROVE UPON FOR THIS COMING WEEK?

If you don't like the story you've been telling yourself, rewrite it.

DAILY CHECK-IN

.... / .... / ....   M   T   W   T   F   S   S

BREAKFAST	
SNACK	
LUNCH	
SNACK	
DINNER	
WORKOUT	
WATER	

WHAT WENT WELL?

WHAT WERE YOUR CHALLENGES?

INSPIRATION FOR TOMORROW:

RATE YOUR DAY

1   2   3   4   5   6   7   8   9   10

DAILY CHECK-IN

.... / .... / ....   M   T   W   T   F   S   S

BREAKFAST	
SNACK	
LUNCH	
SNACK	
DINNER	
WORKOUT	
WATER	

WHAT WENT WELL?

WHAT WERE YOUR CHALLENGES?

INSPIRATION FOR TOMORROW:

RATE YOUR DAY

1   2   3   4   5   6   7   8   9   10

.... / .... / ....   M   T   W   T   F   S   S

BREAKFAST	
SNACK	
LUNCH	
SNACK	
DINNER	
WORKOUT	
WATER	

WHAT WENT WELL?

WHAT WERE YOUR CHALLENGES?

INSPIRATION FOR TOMORROW:

RATE YOUR DAY

1   2   3   4   5   6   7   8   9   10

.... / .... / ....   M   T   W   T   F   S   S

BREAKFAST	
SNACK	
LUNCH	
SNACK	
DINNER	
WORKOUT	
WATER	

WHAT WENT WELL?

WHAT WERE YOUR CHALLENGES?

INSPIRATION FOR TOMORROW:

RATE YOUR DAY

1   2   3   4   5   6   7   8   9   10

DAILY CHECK-IN

.... / .... / .... M T W T F S S

	WHAT WENT WELL?
BREAKFAST	
SNACK	
LUNCH	WHAT WERE YOUR CHALLENGES?
SNACK	
DINNER	INSPIRATION FOR TOMORROW:
WORKOUT	
WATER	RATE YOUR DAY 1 2 3 4 5 6 7 8 9 10

DAILY CHECK-IN

.... / .... / .... M T W T F S S

	WHAT WENT WELL?
BREAKFAST	
SNACK	
LUNCH	WHAT WERE YOUR CHALLENGES?
SNACK	
DINNER	INSPIRATION FOR TOMORROW:
WORKOUT	
WATER	RATE YOUR DAY 1 2 3 4 5 6 7 8 9 10

_____ / _____ / _____   M T W T F S S

| BREAKFAST |
| SNACK |
| LUNCH |
| SNACK |
| DINNER |
| WORKOUT |
| WATER |

WHAT WENT WELL?

WHAT WERE YOUR CHALLENGES?

INSPIRATION FOR TOMORROW:

RATE YOUR DAY

1   2   3   4   5   6   7   8   9   10

YOU CAN'T MEASURE WHAT YOU DON'T TRACK

FROM ___ / ___ / ___ TO___ / ___ / ___

PROGRESS PIC

PROGRESS PIC

STATS

	MEASURE	LOSS/GAIN		MEASURE	LOSS/GAIN
BUST			L HIGH		
WAIST			R ARM		
HIPS			L ARM		
R THIGH			WEIGHT		

MIND MAP

WHAT DO YOU HAVE TO OVERCOME THIS WEEK?

....

....

....

....

RATE YOUR
DEDICATION

ON A SCALE OF 1 TO 10

MENTAL FOCUS	1	2	3	4	5	6	7	8	9	10
COMMITMENT	1	2	3	4	5	6	7	8	9	10
DIET	1	2	3	4	5	6	7	8	9	10
EXERCISE	1	2	3	4	5	6	7	8	9	10

PLAN FOR SUCCESS

CONTROLLABLES VS NON-CONTROLLABLES

CONTROLS 1=Y 0=N	S	M	T	W	TH	F	S	TOTAL
1 (DIET)								
2 (DIET)								
3 (DIET)								
1 (EXERCISE)								
2 (EXERCISE)								
1 (NON-CONTROLLABLE)								

MAKE IT HAPPEN

PREPARATION	GOALS
MEAL PREP	MILESTONE 1
SCHEDULE DIET CONTROLS	MILESTONE 2
SCHEDULE MOVEMENT CONTROLS	MILESTONE 3

WHAT CAN YOU IMPROVE UPON FOR THIS COMING WEEK?

When it would be easier to stay stuck, you must decide to keep moving.

DAILY CHECK-IN

.... / .... / ....   M   T   W   T   F   S   S

BREAKFAST	
SNACK	
LUNCH	
SNACK	
DINNER	
WORKOUT	
WATER	

WHAT WENT WELL?

WHAT WERE YOUR CHALLENGES?

INSPIRATION FOR TOMORROW:

RATE YOUR DAY

1   2   3   4   5   6   7   8   9   10

DAILY CHECK-IN

.... / .... / ....   M   T   W   T   F   S   S

BREAKFAST	
SNACK	
LUNCH	
SNACK	
DINNER	
WORKOUT	
WATER	

WHAT WENT WELL?

WHAT WERE YOUR CHALLENGES?

INSPIRATION FOR TOMORROW:

RATE YOUR DAY

1   2   3   4   5   6   7   8   9   10

.... / .... / ....   M   T   W   T   F   S   S

	WHAT WENT WELL?
BREAKFAST	
SNACK	
LUNCH	WHAT WERE YOUR CHALLENGES?
SNACK	
DINNER	INSPIRATION FOR TOMORROW:
WORKOUT	
WATER	RATE YOUR DAY 1 2 3 4 5 6 7 8 9 10

.... / .... / ....   M   T   W   T   F   S   S

	WHAT WENT WELL?
BREAKFAST	
SNACK	
LUNCH	WHAT WERE YOUR CHALLENGES?
SNACK	
DINNER	INSPIRATION FOR TOMORROW:
WORKOUT	
WATER	RATE YOUR DAY 1 2 3 4 5 6 7 8 9 10

DAILY CHECK-IN

.... / .... / ....   M T W T F S S

BREAKFAST	
SNACK	
LUNCH	
SNACK	
DINNER	
WORKOUT	
WATER	

WHAT WENT WELL?

WHAT WERE YOUR CHALLENGES?

INSPIRATION FOR TOMORROW:

RATE YOUR DAY

1   2   3   4   5   6   7   8   9   10

DAILY CHECK-IN

.... / .... / ....   M T W T F S S

BREAKFAST	
SNACK	
LUNCH	
SNACK	
DINNER	
WORKOUT	
WATER	

WHAT WENT WELL?

WHAT WERE YOUR CHALLENGES?

INSPIRATION FOR TOMORROW:

RATE YOUR DAY

1   2   3   4   5   6   7   8   9   10

_____ / _____ / _____   M T W T F S S

BREAKFAST
SNACK
LUNCH
SNACK
DINNER
WORKOUT
WATER

WHAT WENT WELL?

WHAT WERE YOUR CHALLENGES?

INSPIRATION FOR TOMORROW:

RATE YOUR DAY

1 2 3 4 5 6 7 8 9 10

YOU CAN'T MEASURE WHAT YOU DON'T TRACK

FROM ___ / ___ / ___ TO ___ / ___ / ___

PROGRESS PIC

PROGRESS PIC

STATS

	MEASURE	LOSS/GAIN		MEASURE	LOSS/GAIN
BUST			L HIGH		
WAIST			R ARM		
HIPS			L ARM		
R THIGH			WEIGHT		

MIND MAP

WHAT DO YOU HAVE TO OVERCOME THIS WEEK?

....

....

....

....

RATE YOUR DEDICATION											
ON A SCALE OF 1 TO 10	MENTAL FOCUS	1	2	3	4	5	6	7	8	9	10
	COMMITMENT	1	2	3	4	5	6	7	8	9	10
	DIET	1	2	3	4	5	6	7	8	9	10
	EXERCISE	1	2	3	4	5	6	7	8	9	10

LET'S REVIEW AND MAKE SOME NEW GOALS

What worked, what didn't, and why.

WHAT'S GONE WELL FOR YOU THIS MONTH?

....

....

....

WHAT ARE SOME WINS YOU'VE EXPERIENCED? REMEMBER, NO WIN IS TOO SMALL!

....

....

....

WHAT ARE SOME AREAS YOU'VE STRUGGLED WITH?

....

....

....

REVIEW YOUR WEEKLY CHECK-INS AND YOUR CONTROLLABLE VS.UNCONTROLLABLE CHART.

....

....

....

WHAT CAN YOU FOCUS ON THIS MONTH TO MAKE SURE YOU CONTINUE TO SEE RESULTS?

....

....

....

HOW DO YOU NEED TO ADJUST YOUR GOALS?

MENTAL GOALS	PHYSICAL GOALS
....	....
....	....
....	....

Month 2

You Are More Than Just A Number

Have you stepped on the scale, been disappointed by the number you saw, and then let it ruin your entire day? Week?

If you are anything like me, you've done it a million times. It may even be part of your daily routine. If it is, I am asking you to please stop today.

There was a time when I weighed myself every single morning. I would wake up, try to make myself as light as possible, take a deep breath and then step on the scale.

When I saw the number, I would think a string of expletives and immediately say awful things to myself. Things I would never think about or say to anyone else and things that are tough to admit now.

THINGS LIKE:

You are so disgusting. What is wrong with you? You know what you need to do to lose weight. Why can't you get it together? Do you want to be fat and disgusting the rest of your life? You fail every single time you try. What's your problem? Millions of people have lost weight. Why can't you? You're such a loser.

I would replay these messages in my head all day long. I was consumed by them. This thinking did not help me. It made me feel more alone and like a failure. It seemed like a never-ending cycle. Finally, I realized that I had to take the emotion out of the scale. I started being kinder to myself and being patient with my progress.

I started to give myself compliments instead of constantly tearing myself down.

I SAID THINGS LIKE:

You have a pretty smile. You're kicking butt! You worked out 5 times this week. You rock! Hmmm... your butt is looking rounder.

In the beginning it was very weird and kind of half-hearted. But then I realized how important it was to recognize my effort and own my successes (no matter the size). I also recognized that it made a huge difference in how I felt about myself and whether or not I was enjoying my journey.

As you go into month two of your transformation journey, focus on being kind to yourself. Recognize and appreciate your wins (no matter the size!).

Remember, the number on the scale does not define your value as a human being. It simply tells you what your body weighs. It can't measure the weight of your kindness, the size of your heart, the sacrifices you have made for those you love, or your incredible potential in life. After all, it's just a number.

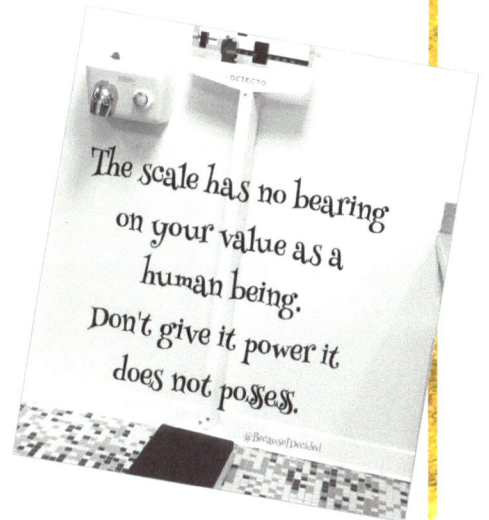

The scale has no bearing on your value as a human being. Don't give it power it does not posses.

@BecauseIDecided

SET YOUR GOALS

Make goals to measure your success.

WHAT IS YOUR MIDSET GOAL FOR THE MONTH?

....

....

....

....

WHAT IS YOUR PHYSICAL GOAL FOR THE MONTH?

....

....

....

....

WHAT DO YOU THINK WILL BE YOUR BIGGEST OBSTACLES?

....

....

....

....

WHAT CAN YOU DO TO SET YOURSELF UP FOR SUCCESS?

....

....

....

....

WHAT IS YOUR PROMISE TO YOURSELF THIS MONTH?

....

....

....

....

WHAT ARE YOUR MILESTONES FOR SUCCESS?

MENTAL MILESTONES   PHYSICAL MILESTONES

....

....

....

CONTROLLABLES VS NON-CONTROLLABLES

CONTROLS 1=Y 0=N	S	M	T	W	TH	F	S	TOTAL
1 (DIET)								
2 (DIET)								
3 (DIET)								
1 (EXERCISE)								
2 (EXERCISE)								
1 (NON-CONTROLLABLE)								

---- MAKE IT HAPPEN ----

PREPARATION

MEAL PREP

SCHEDULE DIET CONTROLS

SCHEDULE MOVEMENT CONTROLS

GOALS

MILESTONE 1

MILESTONE 2

MILESTONE 3

WHAT CAN YOU IMPROVE UPON FOR THIS COMING WEEK?

Talk to yourself like you would to someone you love.

DAILY CHECK-IN

.... / .... / ....   M T W T F S S

BREAKFAST
SNACK
LUNCH
SNACK
DINNER
WORKOUT
WATER

WHAT WENT WELL?

WHAT WERE YOUR CHALLENGES?

INSPIRATION FOR TOMORROW:

RATE YOUR DAY

1   2   3   4   5   6   7   8   9   10

DAILY CHECK-IN

.... / .... / ....   M T W T F S S

BREAKFAST
SNACK
LUNCH
SNACK
DINNER
WORKOUT
WATER

WHAT WENT WELL?

WHAT WERE YOUR CHALLENGES?

INSPIRATION FOR TOMORROW:

RATE YOUR DAY

1   2   3   4   5   6   7   8   9   10

.... / .... / ....   M   T   W   T   F   S   S

| BREAKFAST |
| SNACK |
| LUNCH |
| SNACK |
| DINNER |
| WORKOUT |
| WATER |

WHAT WENT WELL?

WHAT WERE YOUR CHALLENGES?

INSPIRATION FOR TOMORROW:

RATE YOUR DAY

1   2   3   4   5   6   7   8   9   10

.... / .... / ....   M   T   W   T   F   S   S

| BREAKFAST |
| SNACK |
| LUNCH |
| SNACK |
| DINNER |
| WORKOUT |
| WATER |

WHAT WENT WELL?

WHAT WERE YOUR CHALLENGES?

INSPIRATION FOR TOMORROW:

RATE YOUR DAY

1   2   3   4   5   6   7   8   9   10

DAILY CHECK-IN

.... / .... / ....   M   T   W   T   F   S   S

	WHAT WENT WELL?
BREAKFAST	
SNACK	
LUNCH	WHAT WERE YOUR CHALLENGES?
SNACK	
DINNER	INSPIRATION FOR TOMORROW:
WORKOUT	
WATER	RATE YOUR DAY
	1 2 3 4 5 6 7 8 9 10

DAILY CHECK-IN

.... / .... / ....   M   T   W   T   F   S   S

	WHAT WENT WELL?
BREAKFAST	
SNACK	
LUNCH	WHAT WERE YOUR CHALLENGES?
SNACK	
DINNER	INSPIRATION FOR TOMORROW:
WORKOUT	
WATER	RATE YOUR DAY
	1 2 3 4 5 6 7 8 9 10

.... / .... / ....   M T W T F S S

BREAKFAST	
SNACK	
LUNCH	
SNACK	
DINNER	
WORKOUT	
WATER	

WHAT WENT WELL?

WHAT WERE YOUR CHALLENGES?

INSPIRATION FOR TOMORROW:

RATE YOUR DAY

1   2   3   4   5   6   7   8   9   10

YOU CAN'T MEASURE WHAT YOU DON'T TRACK

FROM ___ / ___ / ___ TO ___ / ___ / ___

PROGRESS PIC	PROGRESS PIC

STATS

	MEASURE	LOSS/GAIN		MEASURE	LOSS/GAIN
BUST			L HIGH		
WAIST			R ARM		
HIPS			L ARM		
R THIGH			WEIGHT		

MIND MAP

WHAT DO YOU HAVE TO OVERCOME THIS WEEK?

....

....

....

....

RATE YOUR DEDICATION
ON A SCALE OF 1 TO 10

MENTAL FOCUS	1	2	3	4	5	6	7	8	9	10
COMMITMENT	1	2	3	4	5	6	7	8	9	10
DIET	1	2	3	4	5	6	7	8	9	10
EXERCISE	1	2	3	4	5	6	7	8	9	10

PLAN FOR SUCCESS

CONTROLLABLES VS NON-CONTROLLABLES

CONTROLS 1=Y 0=N	S	M	T	W	TH	F	S	TOTAL
1 (DIET)								
2 (DIET)								
3 (DIET)								
1 (EXERCISE)								
2 (EXERCISE)								
1 (NON-CONTROLLABLE)								

- - - - - - - - - - - - - - MAKE IT HAPPEN - - - - - - - - - - - - - -

PREPARATION	GOALS
MEAL PREP	MILESTONE 1
SCHEDULE DIET CONTROLS	MILESTONE 2
SCHEDULE MOVEMENT CONTROLS	MILESTONE 3

WHAT CAN YOU IMPROVE UPON FOR THIS COMING WEEK?

*Beautiful girl,
you can do
incredible things.*

DAILY CHECK-IN

.... / .... / ....   M   T   W   T   F   S   S

BREAKFAST	
SNACK	
LUNCH	
SNACK	
DINNER	
WORKOUT	
WATER	

WHAT WENT WELL?

WHAT WERE YOUR CHALLENGES?

INSPIRATION FOR TOMORROW:

RATE YOUR DAY

1   2   3   4   5   6   7   8   9   10

DAILY CHECK-IN

.... / .... / ....   M   T   W   T   F   S   S

BREAKFAST	
SNACK	
LUNCH	
SNACK	
DINNER	
WORKOUT	
WATER	

WHAT WENT WELL?

WHAT WERE YOUR CHALLENGES?

INSPIRATION FOR TOMORROW:

RATE YOUR DAY

1   2   3   4   5   6   7   8   9   10

.... / .... / ....   M   T   W   T   F   S   S

| BREAKFAST |
| SNACK |
| LUNCH |
| SNACK |
| DINNER |
| WORKOUT |
| WATER |

WHAT WENT WELL?

WHAT WERE YOUR CHALLENGES?

INSPIRATION FOR TOMORROW:

RATE YOUR DAY

1   2   3   4   5   6   7   8   9   10

.... / .... / ....   M   T   W   T   F   S   S

| BREAKFAST |
| SNACK |
| LUNCH |
| SNACK |
| DINNER |
| WORKOUT |
| WATER |

WHAT WENT WELL?

WHAT WERE YOUR CHALLENGES?

INSPIRATION FOR TOMORROW:

RATE YOUR DAY

1   2   3   4   5   6   7   8   9   10

DAILY CHECK-IN

.... / .... / ....   M T W T F S S

BREAKFAST

SNACK

LUNCH

SNACK

DINNER

WORKOUT

WATER

WHAT WENT WELL?

WHAT WERE YOUR CHALLENGES?

INSPIRATION FOR TOMORROW:

RATE YOUR DAY

1 2 3 4 5 6 7 8 9 10

DAILY CHECK-IN

.... / .... / ....   M T W T F S S

BREAKFAST

SNACK

LUNCH

SNACK

DINNER

WORKOUT

WATER

WHAT WENT WELL?

WHAT WERE YOUR CHALLENGES?

INSPIRATION FOR TOMORROW:

RATE YOUR DAY

1 2 3 4 5 6 7 8 9 10

.... / .... / ....   M   T   W   T   F   S   S

BREAKFAST	
SNACK	
LUNCH	
SNACK	
DINNER	
WORKOUT	
WATER	

WHAT WENT WELL?

WHAT WERE YOUR CHALLENGES?

INSPIRATION FOR TOMORROW:

RATE YOUR DAY

1   2   3   4   5   6   7   8   9   10

YOU CAN'T MEASURE WHAT YOU DON'T TRACK

FROM ___ / ___ / ___   TO ___ / ___ / ___

PROGRESS PIC	PROGRESS PIC

STATS

	MEASURE	LOSS/GAIN		MEASURE	LOSS/GAIN
BUST			L HIGH		
WAIST			R ARM		
HIPS			L ARM		
R THIGH			WEIGHT		

MIND MAP

WHAT DO YOU HAVE TO OVERCOME THIS WEEK?

....
....
....
....

RATE YOUR DEDICATION — ON A SCALE OF 1 TO 10											
MENTAL FOCUS	1	2	3	4	5	6	7	8	9	10	
COMMITMENT	1	2	3	4	5	6	7	8	9	10	
DIET	1	2	3	4	5	6	7	8	9	10	
EXERCISE	1	2	3	4	5	6	7	8	9	10	

PLAN FOR SUCCESS

CONTROLLABLES VS NON-CONTROLLABLES

CONTROLS 1=Y 0=N	S	M	T	W	TH	F	S	TOTAL
1 (DIET)								
2 (DIET)								
3 (DIET)								
1 (EXERCISE)								
2 (EXERCISE)								
1 (NON-CONTROLLABLE)								

- - - - - - - - - - - - - - - - - MAKE IT HAPPEN - - - - - - - - - - - - - - - - -

PREPARATION

MEAL PREP

SCHEDULE DIET CONTROLS

SCHEDULE MOVEMENT CONTROLS

GOALS

MILESTONE 1

MILESTONE 2

MILESTONE 3

WHAT CAN YOU IMPROVE UPON FOR THIS COMING WEEK?

Always be a work in progress.

DAILY CHECK-IN

.... / .... / ....   M T W T F S S

BREAKFAST	
SNACK	
LUNCH	
SNACK	
DINNER	
WORKOUT	
WATER	

WHAT WENT WELL?

WHAT WERE YOUR CHALLENGES?

INSPIRATION FOR TOMORROW:

RATE YOUR DAY

1   2   3   4   5   6   7   8   9   10

DAILY CHECK-IN

.... / .... / ....   M T W T F S S

BREAKFAST	
SNACK	
LUNCH	
SNACK	
DINNER	
WORKOUT	
WATER	

WHAT WENT WELL?

WHAT WERE YOUR CHALLENGES?

INSPIRATION FOR TOMORROW:

RATE YOUR DAY

1   2   3   4   5   6   7   8   9   10

_____ / _____ / _____　　M　T　W　T　F　S　S

| BREAKFAST |
| SNACK |
| LUNCH |
| SNACK |
| DINNER |
| WORKOUT |
| WATER |

WHAT WENT WELL?

WHAT WERE YOUR CHALLENGES?

INSPIRATION FOR TOMORROW:

RATE YOUR DAY

1　2　3　4　5　6　7　8　9　10

_____ / _____ / _____　　M　T　W　T　F　S　S

| BREAKFAST |
| SNACK |
| LUNCH |
| SNACK |
| DINNER |
| WORKOUT |
| WATER |

WHAT WENT WELL?

WHAT WERE YOUR CHALLENGES?

INSPIRATION FOR TOMORROW:

RATE YOUR DAY

1　2　3　4　5　6　7　8　9　10

.... / .... / ....   M   T   W   T   F   S   S

BREAKFAST	
SNACK	
LUNCH	
SNACK	
DINNER	
WORKOUT	
WATER	

WHAT WENT WELL?

WHAT WERE YOUR CHALLENGES?

INSPIRATION FOR TOMORROW:

RATE YOUR DAY

1   2   3   4   5   6   7   8   9   10

DAILY CHECK-IN

.... / .... / ....   M   T   W   T   F   S   S

BREAKFAST	
SNACK	
LUNCH	
SNACK	
DINNER	
WORKOUT	
WATER	

WHAT WENT WELL?

WHAT WERE YOUR CHALLENGES?

INSPIRATION FOR TOMORROW:

RATE YOUR DAY

1   2   3   4   5   6   7   8   9   10

.... / .... / ....   M T W T F S S

| BREAKFAST |
| SNACK |
| LUNCH |
| SNACK |
| DINNER |
| WORKOUT |
| WATER |

WHAT WENT WELL?

WHAT WERE YOUR CHALLENGES?

INSPIRATION FOR TOMORROW:

RATE YOUR DAY

1   2   3   4   5   6   7   8   9   10

YOU CAN'T MEASURE WHAT YOU DON'T TRACK

FROM ___ / ___ / ___ TO ___ / ___ / ___

PROGRESS PIC

PROGRESS PIC

STATS

	MEASURE	LOSS/GAIN		MEASURE	LOSS/GAIN
BUST			L HIGH		
WAIST			R ARM		
HIPS			L ARM		
R THIGH			WEIGHT		

MIND MAP

WHAT DO YOU HAVE TO OVERCOME THIS WEEK?

....

....

....

....

RATE YOUR DEDICATION

ON A SCALE OF 1 TO 10

MENTAL FOCUS	1	2	3	4	5	6	7	8	9	10
COMMITMENT	1	2	3	4	5	6	7	8	9	10
DIET	1	2	3	4	5	6	7	8	9	10
EXERCISE	1	2	3	4	5	6	7	8	9	10

PLAN FOR SUCCESS

CONTROLLABLES VS NON-CONTROLLABLES

CONTROLS 1=Y 0=N	S	M	T	W	TH	F	S	TOTAL
1 (DIET)								
2 (DIET)								
3 (DIET)								
1 (EXERCISE)								
2 (EXERCISE)								
1 (NON-CONTROLLABLE)								

- - - - - - - MAKE IT HAPPEN - - - - - - -

PREPARATION	GOALS
MEAL PREP	MILESTONE 1
SCHEDULE DIET CONTROLS	MILESTONE 2
SCHEDULE MOVEMENT CONTROLS	MILESTONE 3

WHAT CAN YOU IMPROVE UPON FOR THIS COMING WEEK?

You can't start the next chapter if you keep re-reading the last one.

DAILY CHECK-IN

.... / .... / .... M T W T F S S

BREAKFAST	
SNACK	
LUNCH	
SNACK	
DINNER	
WORKOUT	
WATER	

WHAT WENT WELL?

WHAT WERE YOUR CHALLENGES?

INSPIRATION FOR TOMORROW:

RATE YOUR DAY

1 2 3 4 5 6 7 8 9 10

DAILY CHECK-IN

.... / .... / .... M T W T F S S

BREAKFAST	
SNACK	
LUNCH	
SNACK	
DINNER	
WORKOUT	
WATER	

WHAT WENT WELL?

WHAT WERE YOUR CHALLENGES?

INSPIRATION FOR TOMORROW:

RATE YOUR DAY

1 2 3 4 5 6 7 8 9 10

.... / .... / ....   M   T   W   T   F   S   S

| BREAKFAST |
| SNACK |
| LUNCH |
| SNACK |
| DINNER |
| WORKOUT |
| WATER |

WHAT WENT WELL?

WHAT WERE YOUR CHALLENGES?

INSPIRATION FOR TOMORROW:

RATE YOUR DAY

1   2   3   4   5   6   7   8   9   10

.... / .... / ....   M   T   W   T   F   S   S

| BREAKFAST |
| SNACK |
| LUNCH |
| SNACK |
| DINNER |
| WORKOUT |
| WATER |

WHAT WENT WELL?

WHAT WERE YOUR CHALLENGES?

INSPIRATION FOR TOMORROW:

RATE YOUR DAY

1   2   3   4   5   6   7   8   9   10

DAILY CHECK-IN

.... / .... / ....   M   T   W   T   F   S   S

BREAKFAST
SNACK
LUNCH
SNACK
DINNER
WORKOUT
WATER

WHAT WENT WELL?

WHAT WERE YOUR CHALLENGES?

INSPIRATION FOR TOMORROW:

RATE YOUR DAY

1   2   3   4   5   6   7   8   9   10

DAILY CHECK-IN

.... / .... / ....   M   T   W   T   F   S   S

BREAKFAST
SNACK
LUNCH
SNACK
DINNER
WORKOUT
WATER

WHAT WENT WELL?

WHAT WERE YOUR CHALLENGES?

INSPIRATION FOR TOMORROW:

RATE YOUR DAY

1   2   3   4   5   6   7   8   9   10

_____ / _____ / _____   M T W T F S S

| BREAKFAST |
| SNACK |
| LUNCH |
| SNACK |
| DINNER |
| WORKOUT |
| WATER |

WHAT WENT WELL?

WHAT WERE YOUR CHALLENGES?

INSPIRATION FOR TOMORROW:

RATE YOUR DAY

1 2 3 4 5 6 7 8 9 10

YOU CAN'T MEASURE WHAT YOU DON'T TRACK

FROM ___ / ___ / ___   TO ___ / ___ / ___

PROGRESS PIC	PROGRESS PIC

STATS

	MEASURE	LOSS/GAIN		MEASURE	LOSS/GAIN
BUST			L HIGH		
WAIST			R ARM		
HIPS			L ARM		
R THIGH			WEIGHT		

MIND MAP

WHAT DO YOU HAVE TO OVERCOME THIS WEEK?

....

....

....

....

RATE YOUR DEDICATION ON A SCALE OF 1 TO 10											
MENTAL FOCUS	1	2	3	4	5	6	7	8	9	10	
COMMITMENT	1	2	3	4	5	6	7	8	9	10	
DIET	1	2	3	4	5	6	7	8	9	10	
EXERCISE	1	2	3	4	5	6	7	8	9	10	

LET'S REVIEW AND MAKE SOME NEW GOALS

What worked, what didn't, and why.

WHAT'S GONE WELL FOR YOU THIS MONTH?

....

....

....

....

WHAT ARE SOME WINS YOU'VE EXPERIENCED? REMEMBER, NO WIN IS TOO SMALL!

....

....

....

....

WHAT ARE SOME AREAS YOU'VE STRUGGLED WITH?

....

....

....

....

REVIEW YOUR WEEKLY CHECK-INS AND YOUR CONTROLLABLE VS.UNCONTROLLABLE CHART.

....

....

....

....

WHAT CAN YOU FOCUS ON THIS MONTH TO MAKE SURE YOU CONTINUE TO SEE RESULTS?

....

....

....

....

HOW DO YOU NEED TO ADJUST YOUR GOALS?

MENTAL GOALS	PHYSICAL GOALS
....	....
....	....
....	....

Month 3

Because I
DECIDED

with Mariah McCullough

When You Feel Like Quitting...

If you give up now, you'll soon be back to where you started. And when you started, you desperately wanted to be where you are today.

When I started out on my transformation journey, I couldn't get up off the floor without rolling onto my side, propping up on my knee, and pushing off a chair or table. I couldn't sleep through the night without having severe back pain and I couldn't shop in a regular-sized clothes store.

I remember feeling weak, incapable, and embarrassed. I longed for the day that I could pop up off the floor like a normal sized person, sleep through the night pain free, and shop in a normal size clothes store.

Six months into my journey I could do all these things. But then I was unhappy because I could barely do a push up on my knees, couldn't do a full sit up, and I had loose skin. I was frustrated because I'd lost a lot of weight but still had so far to go.

I thought about quitting; about going to back to binge eating and being lazy. Then I remembered how desperately I wanted to be able jump up off the floor, sleep pain-free, and wear normal sized clothes.

I decided that I wasn't going back to not being able to do those things. I also decided that no matter how long it took, I was going to keep working until I could do regular push-ups and sit ups. I didn't know if I'd ever lose my loose skin, but I wasn't going to let it stop me from moving forward.

Now, 10 years later, I can knock out multiple sets of 20 regular push-ups, countless sit ups, and my loose skin has tightened. It didn't happen overnight. The changes came because of what I did daily. I consistently put work in and took care of myself.

If I'd quit every time I got discouraged, then you wouldn't be reading this today because I would have given up on myself and likely would have returned to the woman who couldn't get off the floor unassisted.

As you go through your transformation journey, there will be times when you feel like quitting because you don't think you're making fast enough progress or because you think you have too far to go.

When you feel like quitting, think about something you can do now that you desperately wanted to be able to do when you started. Use that as motivation to keep moving forward.

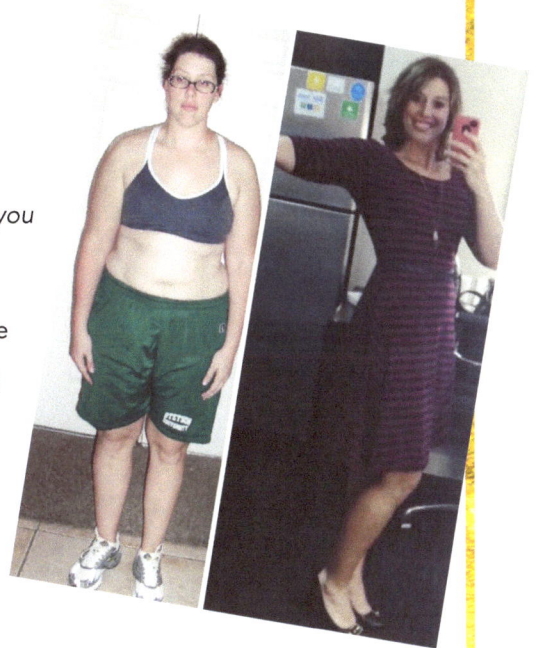

WHAT IS THAT SOMETHING? _____

WHAT IS SOMETHING YOU WISH YOU COULD DO NOW THAT YOU WILL CELEBRATE ONCE YOU CAN DO IT?

_____

SET YOUR GOALS

Make goals to measure your success.

WHAT IS YOUR MIDSET GOAL FOR THE MONTH?

....
....
....
....

WHAT IS YOUR PHYSICAL GOAL FOR THE MONTH?

....
....
....
....

WHAT DO YOU THINK WILL BE YOUR BIGGEST OBSTACLES?

....
....
....
....

WHAT CAN YOU DO TO SET YOURSELF UP FOR SUCCESS?

....
....
....
....

WHAT IS YOUR PROMISE TO YOURSELF THIS MONTH?

....
....
....
....

WHAT ARE YOUR MILESTONES FOR SUCCESS?

MENTAL MILESTONES	PHYSICAL MILESTONES
....	....
....	....
....	....

PLAN FOR SUCCESS

CONTROLLABLES VS NON-CONTROLLABLES

CONTROLS 1=Y 0=N	S	M	T	W	TH	F	S	TOTAL
1 (DIET)								
2 (DIET)								
3 (DIET)								
1 (EXERCISE)								
2 (EXERCISE)								
1 (NON-CONTROLLABLE)								

-------------------------------- MAKE IT HAPPEN --------------------------------

PREPARATION	GOALS
MEAL PREP	MILESTONE 1
SCHEDULE DIET CONTROLS	MILESTONE 2
SCHEDULE MOVEMENT CONTROLS	MILESTONE 3

WHAT CAN YOU IMPROVE UPON FOR THIS COMING WEEK?

Something will grow from all you are going through and it will be YOU.

FOLLOW ME: f P Because_I_Decided   Because_I_Decided

DAILY CHECK-IN

.... / .... / ....   M   T   W   T   F   S   S

BREAKFAST	
SNACK	
LUNCH	
SNACK	
DINNER	
WORKOUT	
WATER	

WHAT WENT WELL?

WHAT WERE YOUR CHALLENGES?

INSPIRATION FOR TOMORROW:

RATE YOUR DAY

1   2   3   4   5   6   7   8   9   10

DAILY CHECK-IN

.... / .... / ....   M   T   W   T   F   S   S

BREAKFAST	
SNACK	
LUNCH	
SNACK	
DINNER	
WORKOUT	
WATER	

WHAT WENT WELL?

WHAT WERE YOUR CHALLENGES?

INSPIRATION FOR TOMORROW:

RATE YOUR DAY

1   2   3   4   5   6   7   8   9   10

.... / .... / ....   M T W T F S S

BREAKFAST	
SNACK	
LUNCH	
SNACK	
DINNER	
WORKOUT	
WATER	

WHAT WENT WELL?

WHAT WERE YOUR CHALLENGES?

INSPIRATION FOR TOMORROW:

RATE YOUR DAY

1   2   3   4   5   6   7   8   9   10

.... / .... / ....   M T W T F S S

BREAKFAST	
SNACK	
LUNCH	
SNACK	
DINNER	
WORKOUT	
WATER	

WHAT WENT WELL?

WHAT WERE YOUR CHALLENGES?

INSPIRATION FOR TOMORROW:

RATE YOUR DAY

1   2   3   4   5   6   7   8   9   10

DAILY CHECK-IN

.... / .... / ....   M T W T F S S

BREAKFAST	
SNACK	
LUNCH	
SNACK	
DINNER	
WORKOUT	
WATER	

WHAT WENT WELL?

WHAT WERE YOUR CHALLENGES?

INSPIRATION FOR TOMORROW:

RATE YOUR DAY

1   2   3   4   5   6   7   8   9   10

DAILY CHECK-IN

.... / .... / ....   M T W T F S S

BREAKFAST	
SNACK	
LUNCH	
SNACK	
DINNER	
WORKOUT	
WATER	

WHAT WENT WELL?

WHAT WERE YOUR CHALLENGES?

INSPIRATION FOR TOMORROW:

RATE YOUR DAY

1   2   3   4   5   6   7   8   9   10

.... / .... / ....   M   T   W   T   F   S   S

BREAKFAST	
SNACK	
LUNCH	
SNACK	
DINNER	
WORKOUT	
WATER	

WHAT WENT WELL?

WHAT WERE YOUR CHALLENGES?

INSPIRATION FOR TOMORROW:

RATE YOUR DAY

1   2   3   4   5   6   7   8   9   10

YOU CAN'T MEASURE WHAT YOU DON'T TRACK

FROM ___ / ___ / ___ TO ___ / ___ / ___

PROGRESS PIC	PROGRESS PIC

STATS

	MEASURE	LOSS/GAIN		MEASURE	LOSS/GAIN
BUST			L HIGH		
WAIST			R ARM		
HIPS			L ARM		
R THIGH			WEIGHT		

MIND MAP

WHAT DO YOU HAVE TO OVERCOME THIS WEEK?

....

....

....

....

RATE YOUR DEDICATION ON A SCALE OF 1 TO 10											
MENTAL FOCUS	1	2	3	4	5	6	7	8	9	10	
COMMITMENT	1	2	3	4	5	6	7	8	9	10	
DIET	1	2	3	4	5	6	7	8	9	10	
EXERCISE	1	2	3	4	5	6	7	8	9	10	

PLAN FOR SUCCESS

CONTROLLABLES VS NON-CONTROLLABLES

CONTROLS 1=Y 0=N	S	M	T	W	TH	F	S	TOTAL
1 (DIET)								
2 (DIET)								
3 (DIET)								
1 (EXERCISE)								
2 (EXERCISE)								
1 (NON-CONTROLLABLE)								

--- MAKE IT HAPPEN ---

PREPARATION	GOALS
MEAL PREP	MILESTONE 1
SCHEDULE DIET CONTROLS	MILESTONE 2
SCHEDULE MOVEMENT CONTROLS	MILESTONE 3

WHAT CAN YOU IMPROVE UPON FOR THIS COMING WEEK?

Become unshake-able in the belief that you are worthy of a big life.

DAILY CHECK-IN

.... / .... / ....   M T W T F S S

BREAKFAST	
SNACK	
LUNCH	
SNACK	
DINNER	
WORKOUT	
WATER	

WHAT WENT WELL?

WHAT WERE YOUR CHALLENGES?

INSPIRATION FOR TOMORROW:

RATE YOUR DAY

1   2   3   4   5   6   7   8   9   10

DAILY CHECK-IN

.... / .... / ....   M T W T F S S

BREAKFAST	
SNACK	
LUNCH	
SNACK	
DINNER	
WORKOUT	
WATER	

WHAT WENT WELL?

WHAT WERE YOUR CHALLENGES?

INSPIRATION FOR TOMORROW:

RATE YOUR DAY

1   2   3   4   5   6   7   8   9   10

.... / .... / ....   M   T   W   T   F   S   S

| BREAKFAST |
| SNACK |
| LUNCH |
| SNACK |
| DINNER |
| WORKOUT |
| WATER |

WHAT WENT WELL?

WHAT WERE YOUR CHALLENGES?

INSPIRATION FOR TOMORROW:

RATE YOUR DAY

1   2   3   4   5   6   7   8   9   10

.... / .... / ....   M   T   W   T   F   S   S

| BREAKFAST |
| SNACK |
| LUNCH |
| SNACK |
| DINNER |
| WORKOUT |
| WATER |

WHAT WENT WELL?

WHAT WERE YOUR CHALLENGES?

INSPIRATION FOR TOMORROW:

RATE YOUR DAY

1   2   3   4   5   6   7   8   9   10

DAILY CHECK-IN

.... / .... / ....   M   T   W   T   F   S   S

BREAKFAST	
SNACK	
LUNCH	
SNACK	
DINNER	
WORKOUT	
WATER	

WHAT WENT WELL?

WHAT WERE YOUR CHALLENGES?

INSPIRATION FOR TOMORROW:

RATE YOUR DAY

1   2   3   4   5   6   7   8   9   10

DAILY CHECK-IN

.... / .... / ....   M   T   W   T   F   S   S

BREAKFAST	
SNACK	
LUNCH	
SNACK	
DINNER	
WORKOUT	
WATER	

WHAT WENT WELL?

WHAT WERE YOUR CHALLENGES?

INSPIRATION FOR TOMORROW:

RATE YOUR DAY

1   2   3   4   5   6   7   8   9   10

.... / .... / ....   M T W T F S S

BREAKFAST	
SNACK	
LUNCH	
SNACK	
DINNER	
WORKOUT	
WATER	

WHAT WENT WELL?

WHAT WERE YOUR CHALLENGES?

INSPIRATION FOR TOMORROW:

RATE YOUR DAY

1   2   3   4   5   6   7   8   9   10

YOU CAN'T MEASURE WHAT YOU DON'T TRACK

FROM ___ / ___ / ___   TO ___ / ___ / ___

| PROGRESS PIC | PROGRESS PIC |

STATS

	MEASURE	LOSS/GAIN		MEASURE	LOSS/GAIN
BUST			L HIGH		
WAIST			R ARM		
HIPS			L ARM		
R THIGH			WEIGHT		

MIND MAP

WHAT DO YOU HAVE TO OVERCOME THIS WEEK?

....

....

....

....

RATE YOUR DEDICATION ON A SCALE OF 1 TO 10											
MENTAL FOCUS	1	2	3	4	5	6	7	8	9	10
COMMITMENT	1	2	3	4	5	6	7	8	9	10
DIET	1	2	3	4	5	6	7	8	9	10
EXERCISE	1	2	3	4	5	6	7	8	9	10

PLAN FOR SUCCESS

CONTROLLABLES VS NON-CONTROLLABLES

CONTROLS 1=Y 0=N	S	M	T	W	TH	F	S	TOTAL
1 (DIET)								
2 (DIET)								
3 (DIET)								
1 (EXERCISE)								
2 (EXERCISE)								
1 (NON-CONTROLLABLE)								

- - - - - - - - - - - - - - - - MAKE IT HAPPEN - - - - - - - - - - - - - - - -

PREPARATION	GOALS
MEAL PREP	MILESTONE 1
SCHEDULE DIET CONTROLS	MILESTONE 2
SCHEDULE MOVEMENT CONTROLS	MILESTONE 3

WHAT CAN YOU IMPROVE UPON FOR THIS COMING WEEK?

She loved life and it loved her back.

FOLLOW ME: f P BecauseIDecided BecauseIDecided

DAILY CHECK-IN

.... / .... / ....   M T W T F S S

BREAKFAST	
SNACK	
LUNCH	
SNACK	
DINNER	
WORKOUT	
WATER	

WHAT WENT WELL?

WHAT WERE YOUR CHALLENGES?

INSPIRATION FOR TOMORROW:

RATE YOUR DAY

1 2 3 4 5 6 7 8 9 10

DAILY CHECK-IN

.... / .... / ....   M T W T F S S

BREAKFAST	
SNACK	
LUNCH	
SNACK	
DINNER	
WORKOUT	
WATER	

WHAT WENT WELL?

WHAT WERE YOUR CHALLENGES?

INSPIRATION FOR TOMORROW:

RATE YOUR DAY

1 2 3 4 5 6 7 8 9 10

.... / .... / ....   M T W T F S S

BREAKFAST	
SNACK	
LUNCH	
SNACK	
DINNER	
WORKOUT	
WATER	

WHAT WENT WELL?

WHAT WERE YOUR CHALLENGES?

INSPIRATION FOR TOMORROW:

RATE YOUR DAY

1   2   3   4   5   6   7   8   9   10

.... / .... / ....   M T W T F S S

BREAKFAST	
SNACK	
LUNCH	
SNACK	
DINNER	
WORKOUT	
WATER	

WHAT WENT WELL?

WHAT WERE YOUR CHALLENGES?

INSPIRATION FOR TOMORROW:

RATE YOUR DAY

1   2   3   4   5   6   7   8   9   10

DAILY CHECK-IN

_____ / _____ / _____   M T W T F S S

BREAKFAST	
SNACK	
LUNCH	
SNACK	
DINNER	
WORKOUT	
WATER	

WHAT WENT WELL?

WHAT WERE YOUR CHALLENGES?

INSPIRATION FOR TOMORROW:

RATE YOUR DAY

1   2   3   4   5   6   7   8   9   10

- -

DAILY CHECK-IN

_____ / _____ / _____   M T W T F S S

BREAKFAST	
SNACK	
LUNCH	
SNACK	
DINNER	
WORKOUT	
WATER	

WHAT WENT WELL?

WHAT WERE YOUR CHALLENGES?

INSPIRATION FOR TOMORROW:

RATE YOUR DAY

1   2   3   4   5   6   7   8   9   10

.... / .... / ....   M T W T F S S

BREAKFAST	
SNACK	
LUNCH	
SNACK	
DINNER	
WORKOUT	
WATER	

WHAT WENT WELL?

WHAT WERE YOUR CHALLENGES?

INSPIRATION FOR TOMORROW:

RATE YOUR DAY

1   2   3   4   5   6   7   8   9   10

YOU CAN'T MEASURE WHAT YOU DON'T TRACK

FROM ___ /___ /___ TO___ /___ /___

PROGRESS PIC

PROGRESS PIC

STATS

	MEASURE	LOSS/GAIN		MEASURE	LOSS/GAIN
BUST			L HIGH		
WAIST			R ARM		
HIPS			L ARM		
R THIGH			WEIGHT		

MIND MAP

WHAT DO YOU HAVE TO OVERCOME THIS WEEK?

....

....

....

....

RATE YOUR
DEDICATION

ON A SCALE OF 1 TO 10

	1	2	3	4	5	6	7	8	9	10
MENTAL FOCUS	1	2	3	4	5	6	7	8	9	10
COMMITMENT	1	2	3	4	5	6	7	8	9	10
DIET	1	2	3	4	5	6	7	8	9	10
EXERCISE	1	2	3	4	5	6	7	8	9	10

PLAN FOR SUCCESS

CONTROLLABLES VS NON-CONTROLLABLES

CONTROLS 1 = Y 0 = N	S	M	T	W	TH	F	S	TOTAL
1 (DIET)								
2 (DIET)								
3 (DIET)								
1 (EXERCISE)								
2 (EXERCISE)								
1 (NON-CONTROLLABLE)								

- - - - - - - - - - - - MAKE IT HAPPEN - - - - - - - - - - - -

PREPARATION	GOALS
MEAL PREP	MILESTONE 1
SCHEDULE DIET CONTROLS	MILESTONE 2
SCHEDULE MOVEMENT CONTROLS	MILESTONE 3

WHAT CAN YOU IMPROVE UPON FOR THIS COMING WEEK?

Just when the caterpillar thought her life was over, she began to fly.

FOLLOW ME: f P BecauseIDecided C Because_I_Decided

DAILY CHECK-IN

.... / .... / ....   M T W T F S S

| BREAKFAST |
| SNACK |
| LUNCH |
| SNACK |
| DINNER |
| WORKOUT |
| WATER |

WHAT WENT WELL?

WHAT WERE YOUR CHALLENGES?

INSPIRATION FOR TOMORROW:

RATE YOUR DAY

1   2   3   4   5   6   7   8   9   10

DAILY CHECK-IN

.... / .... / ....   M T W T F S S

| BREAKFAST |
| SNACK |
| LUNCH |
| SNACK |
| DINNER |
| WORKOUT |
| WATER |

WHAT WENT WELL?

WHAT WERE YOUR CHALLENGES?

INSPIRATION FOR TOMORROW:

RATE YOUR DAY

1   2   3   4   5   6   7   8   9   10

.... / .... / ....   M T W T F S S

BREAKFAST	
SNACK	
LUNCH	
SNACK	
DINNER	
WORKOUT	
WATER	

WHAT WENT WELL?

WHAT WERE YOUR CHALLENGES?

INSPIRATION FOR TOMORROW:

RATE YOUR DAY

1 2 3 4 5 6 7 8 9 10

.... / .... / ....   M T W T F S S

BREAKFAST	
SNACK	
LUNCH	
SNACK	
DINNER	
WORKOUT	
WATER	

WHAT WENT WELL?

WHAT WERE YOUR CHALLENGES?

INSPIRATION FOR TOMORROW:

RATE YOUR DAY

1 2 3 4 5 6 7 8 9 10

DAILY CHECK-IN

.... / .... / ....   M   T   W   T   F   S   S

BREAKFAST	
SNACK	
LUNCH	
SNACK	
DINNER	
WORKOUT	
WATER	

WHAT WENT WELL?

WHAT WERE YOUR CHALLENGES?

INSPIRATION FOR TOMORROW:

RATE YOUR DAY

1   2   3   4   5   6   7   8   9   10

DAILY CHECK-IN

.... / .... / ....   M   T   W   T   F   S   S

BREAKFAST	
SNACK	
LUNCH	
SNACK	
DINNER	
WORKOUT	
WATER	

WHAT WENT WELL?

WHAT WERE YOUR CHALLENGES?

INSPIRATION FOR TOMORROW:

RATE YOUR DAY

1   2   3   4   5   6   7   8   9   10

.... / .... / ....   M T W T F S S

BREAKFAST	
SNACK	
LUNCH	
SNACK	
DINNER	
WORKOUT	
WATER	

WHAT WENT WELL?

WHAT WERE YOUR CHALLENGES?

INSPIRATION FOR TOMORROW:

RATE YOUR DAY

1   2   3   4   5   6   7   8   9   10

YOU CAN'T MEASURE WHAT YOU DON'T TRACK

FROM ___ / ___ / ___   TO ___ / ___ / ___

| | | PROGRESS PIC | | | PROGRESS PIC | |

STATS

	MEASURE	LOSS/GAIN		MEASURE	LOSS/GAIN
BUST			L HIGH		
WAIST			R ARM		
HIPS			L ARM		
R THIGH			WEIGHT		

MIND MAP

WHAT DO YOU HAVE TO OVERCOME THIS WEEK?

....
....
....
....

RATE YOUR DEDICATION											
MENTAL FOCUS	1	2	3	4	5	6	7	8	9	10	
COMMITMENT	1	2	3	4	5	6	7	8	9	10	
DIET	1	2	3	4	5	6	7	8	9	10	
EXERCISE	1	2	3	4	5	6	7	8	9	10	

RATE YOUR DEDICATION — ON A SCALE OF 1 TO 10

PLAN FOR SUCCESS

CONTROLLABLES VS NON-CONTROLLABLES

CONTROLS 1=Y 0=N	S	M	T	W	TH	F	S	TOTAL
1 (DIET)								
2 (DIET)								
3 (DIET)								
1 (EXERCISE)								
2 (EXERCISE)								
1 (NON-CONTROLLABLE)								

- - - - - - - - - - - - - - - MAKE IT HAPPEN - - - - - - - - - - - - - - -

PREPARATION

MEAL PREP

SCHEDULE DIET CONTROLS

SCHEDULE MOVEMENT CONTROLS

GOALS

MILESTONE 1

MILESTONE 2

MILESTONE 3

WHAT CAN YOU IMPROVE UPON FOR THIS COMING WEEK?

Only you can control your future.

DAILY CHECK-IN

.... / .... / ....   M T W T F S S

BREAKFAST

SNACK

LUNCH

SNACK

DINNER

WORKOUT

WATER

WHAT WENT WELL?

WHAT WERE YOUR CHALLENGES?

INSPIRATION FOR TOMORROW:

RATE YOUR DAY

1 2 3 4 5 6 7 8 9 10

DAILY CHECK-IN

.... / .... / ....   M T W T F S S

BREAKFAST

SNACK

LUNCH

SNACK

DINNER

WORKOUT

WATER

WHAT WENT WELL?

WHAT WERE YOUR CHALLENGES?

INSPIRATION FOR TOMORROW:

RATE YOUR DAY

1 2 3 4 5 6 7 8 9 10

.... / .... / ....   M   T   W   T   F   S   S

| BREAKFAST |
| SNACK |
| LUNCH |
| SNACK |
| DINNER |
| WORKOUT |
| WATER |

WHAT WENT WELL?

WHAT WERE YOUR CHALLENGES?

INSPIRATION FOR TOMORROW:

RATE YOUR DAY

1   2   3   4   5   6   7   8   9   10

.... / .... / ....   M   T   W   T   F   S   S

| BREAKFAST |
| SNACK |
| LUNCH |
| SNACK |
| DINNER |
| WORKOUT |
| WATER |

WHAT WENT WELL?

WHAT WERE YOUR CHALLENGES?

INSPIRATION FOR TOMORROW:

RATE YOUR DAY

1   2   3   4   5   6   7   8   9   10

DAILY CHECK-IN

.... / .... / ....   M T W T F S S

BREAKFAST	
SNACK	
LUNCH	
SNACK	
DINNER	
WORKOUT	
WATER	

WHAT WENT WELL?

WHAT WERE YOUR CHALLENGES?

INSPIRATION FOR TOMORROW:

RATE YOUR DAY

1   2   3   4   5   6   7   8   9   10

DAILY CHECK-IN

.... / .... / ....   M T W T F S S

BREAKFAST	
SNACK	
LUNCH	
SNACK	
DINNER	
WORKOUT	
WATER	

WHAT WENT WELL?

WHAT WERE YOUR CHALLENGES?

INSPIRATION FOR TOMORROW:

RATE YOUR DAY

1   2   3   4   5   6   7   8   9   10

.... / .... / ....   M T W T F S S

SNACK

LUNCH

SNACK

DINNER

WORKOUT

WATER

WHAT WENT WELL?

WHAT WERE YOUR CHALLENGES?

INSPIRATION FOR TOMORROW:

RATE YOUR DAY

1   2   3   4   5   6   7   8   9   10

REFLECTION

YOU CAN'T MEASURE WHAT YOU DON'T TRACK

FROM ___ / ___ / ___ TO ___ / ___ / ___

PROGRESS PIC	PROGRESS PIC

STATS

	MEASURE	LOSS/GAIN		MEASURE	LOSS/GAIN
BUST			L HIGH		
WAIST			R ARM		
HIPS			L ARM		
R THIGH			WEIGHT		

MIND MAP

WHAT DO YOU HAVE TO OVERCOME THIS WEEK?

....

....

....

....

RATE YOUR DEDICATION
ON A SCALE OF 1 TO 10

MENTAL FOCUS	1	2	3	4	5	6	7	8	9	10
COMMITMENT	1	2	3	4	5	6	7	8	9	10
DIET	1	2	3	4	5	6	7	8	9	10
EXERCISE	1	2	3	4	5	6	7	8	9	10

LET'S REVIEW AND MAKE SOME NEW GOALS

What worked, what didn't, and why.

WHAT'S GONE WELL FOR YOU THIS MONTH?

....

....

....

....

WHAT ARE SOME WINS YOU'VE EXPERIENCED? REMEMBER, NO WIN IS TOO SMALL!

....

....

....

WHAT ARE SOME AREAS YOU'VE STRUGGLED WITH?

....

....

....

REVIEW YOUR WEEKLY CHECK-INS AND YOUR CONTROLLABLE VS.UNCONTROLLABLE CHART.

....

....

....

WHAT CAN YOU FOCUS ON THIS MONTH TO MAKE SURE YOU CONTINUE TO SEE RESULTS?

....

....

....

HOW DO YOU NEED TO ADJUST YOUR GOALS?

MENTAL GOALS	PHYSICAL GOALS
....	....
....	....
....	....

You Did It!

WHAT'S NEXT?

Because I
DECIDED

with Mariah McCullough

TIME TO CELEBRATE

FROM ___ / ___ / ___   TO ___ / ___ / ___

PROGRESS PIC
BEFORE

PROGRESS PIC
AFTER

STATS

	START	END	LOSS/GAIN
BUST			
WAIST			
HIPS			
R THIGH			

	START	END	LOSS/GAIN
L HIGH			
R ARM			
L ARM			
WEIGHT			

Woooohooo! You did it. YOU DID IT!

Throughout the journal, you'll find tips, tricks and strategies sprinkled on the pages. These are things that I've used along my journey that you may find helpful on yours. Use the ones that work for you and forget about the ones that aren't appealing to you. Remember, this is your journey and you have to make tips, tricks and strategies work for you.

HOW AM I DIFFERENT NOW THAN I WAS 90 DAYS AGO?

WHAT CHALLENGES DID I OVERCOME TO MAKE IT HERE?

WHAT DID I LEARN ABOUT MYSELF?

IF I COULD GO BACK IN TIME 90 DAYS, WHAT WOULD I TELL MYSELF THAT WOULD MAKE THE 90 DAYS EASIER OR MORE ENJOYABLE?

....

....

....

....

....

WHAT WAS MY FAVORITE THING ABOUT THIS JOURNEY?

....

....

....

....

....

....

WHAT WAS THE MOST DIFFICULT THING FOR ME ABOUT THIS JOURNEY?

....

....

....

....

....

....

AM I DONE TRANSFORMING OR AM I JUST GETTING STARTED?

....

....

....

....

....

I'm willing to share my answers to these questions and/or my transformation pictures with Mariah McCullough (the creator of this program) so she can celebrate with me! If yes, please either email your answers to Mariah@BecauseIDecided.com or share your responseson Facebook or Instagram and tag @Because_I_Decided.

www.ingramcontent.com/pod-product-compliance
Lightning Source LLC
Chambersburg PA
CBHW060804270326
41927CB00002B/40

9 781732 180307